Medical Assistant Certification Study Guide

Vol 2

Medical Assistant Exam Book

Jane John-Nwankwo   RN, MSN

MEDICAL ASSISTANT CERTIFICATION STUDY GUIDE :
Medical Assistant Exam Book

Vol 2

ISBN-13: 978-1497568730

ISBN-10: 1497568730

Printed in the United States of America.

Dedication

To my loving son, Chidike John(Jr) Nwankwo

OTHER TITLES FROM THE SAME AUTHOR:

1. Work At Home Jobs For Nurses & Other Healthcare Professionals

2. Nurses' Romance Series

3. CNA Exam Prep: Nurse Assistant Practice Test Questions. Vol. One and Two

4. Patient Care Technician Exam Review Questions: PCT Test Prep

5. Accept Challenges

6. Medical Assistant Exam Review

7. Hightime You Made A Move!

8. Phlebotomy Test Prep Vol 1, 2, & 3

9. The Home Health Aide Textbook

10. Workbook for The Home Health Aide Textbook

And Many More Books

Visit www.healthcarepracticetest.com

TABLE OF CONTENTS

Section One

General Information For The Medical Assistant

Urinalysis Section

This department performs physical, chemical, and microscopic examination of urine. The physical examination assesses the color, clarity, and specific gravity of the specimen. Chemical evaluation is done using chemical reagent strips to screen for substances such as sugar and protein. Microscopic examination is done to detect presence of blood cells, bacteria and other substances. Requested cultures are sent to the microbiology department.

The Microscope

One of the most commonly used instruments in the medical laboratory is the compound microscope also known as the bright-field microscope. It has two different lenses and light passes through the specimen and lenses to the observer's eye. Lens on the eyepiece (ocular) compounds or increases the magnification produced of an image by the other lens (objective). Magnification is determined by multiplying the magnifying power of the ocular lens (10X) by the magnifying power of the objective lens (10X, 40X, 100X). The objectives are mounted on a nosepiece which pivots to allow the lenses to rotate. Objective lenses are rated according to focal length (usually, 16-mm, 4-mm, and 1.8-mm) which is the distance from the object examined to the center of the lens. The greater the magnification of the lens, the lesser is the distance between the bottom of the lens and the material viewed.

Low power objective (16-mm, 10X)

This allows the item being viewed to be magnified ten times larger than life. This magnification multiplied with the magnification of the ocular lens allows us to see microscopically one hundred times the normal size (10X x 10X = 100X). This is used for light adjustment, for initial focusing and scanning a subject (e.g. observing the morphology of microorganisms).

High power objective (4-mm, 40X)

By combining the ten-power (10X) ocular lens with the magnification power of forty times life40X), the magnification vision is increased to four hundred times the normal size (10X x 40X = 400X). This is used to view urinary sediments in detail, KOH prep for fungi, and wet mounts for parasites.

Oil immersion objective (1.8-mm, 100X)

This objective enables us to reach a possible total magnification of one thousand times normal life size by multiplying the ocular lens magnification (10X) by one hundred (100X), (10X x 100X = 1,000X). Since more light is needed to actually see this amount of magnification, the lens is immersed in oil. Oil slows down the speed at which light travels preventing the scattering or loss of light rays which naturally occurs when light travels through air. Consequently, the efficiency of the magnification is increased.

This objective is used for observing bacteria, for WBC differential count and RBC morphology

Understanding Laboratory Measurements

Basic Units of the System

Meter

The meter is the basic unit of length. A meter is 39.37 inches long. A decimeter would be 3.94 inches long. A centimeter would be about 0.39 inches long, and a millimeter would be about 0.04 inches in length. One thousand meters would equal 1 km. Meters are often used in laboratory reports, charts, and other data requiring linear measurements. For instance, a laboratory procedure might require you to —connect flasks using 0.3 meters of rubber tubing;‖ this would mean that you must use 12 inches of tubing.

Liter

The liter is the basic unit of capacity or volume. This measure tells us how much space an item occupies. The standard unit for capacity in the International System is expressed in terms of multiples or decimal fractions of the cubic meter. In the laboratory, this unit is too large for everyday use; thus the cubic decimeter is used. The liter is accepted as a general designation for 1 cubic decimeter. The liter is used most frequently in the United States by the beverage industry. We are all familiar with the 2-liter soft drink container. A liter is slightly more than 1 qt and is equal to 1000 mL, or the capacity occupied by 2.2 lb of distilled water at 39.2*C.

Gram

The gram is the basic unit of weight or mass. A measure of weight tells how heavy an item is. One thousand cubic centimeters, the equivalent of 1 cubic decimeter, have the capacity of 1 L and weigh 1000 gm or 1 kg. The kilogram is the standard unit of weight and is equivalent to approximately 2.2 lb in the English system of measurement. In the clinical laboratory, the gram (0.001 kg) is used more frequently than is the kilogram. A gram is the weight of 1 cubic centimeter of distilled water at a temperature of 39.2*C.

Metric Abbreviations

Metric Unit Abbreviation Meter Liter Gram

Meter M(m)

Liter L (l)

Gram g or gm

Kilo k km kL kg

Hecto h hm hL hg

Deca da dam daL dag

Deci d dm mL dg

Centi c cm cL cg

Milli m mm mL mg

Micro u um uL ug

Nano n nm nL ng

Commonly Used Metric Prefixes

Kilo= 1000.00 (One-thousand)

Deci= 0.1 (one-tenth)

Centi= 0.01 (one-hundredth)

Milli= 0.001 (one-thousandth)

Micro= 0.000,001 (one millionth)

Nano= 0.000,000,001 (one billionth)

Solutions and Dilutions

It is necessary to make dilutions in the laboratory frequently. For example, blood, serum, or plasma is diluted to produce color reactions that can be used in determining test results. When blood cell counts are done manually, it is necessary to make a dilution before these cells can be counted under the microscope.

Today, most solutions are commercially prepared and come to the laboratory in a ready-to use package. You know that a 10% bleach solution is the solution of choice in cleaning areas where there is the possibility of body fluid contamination. There will be a time that you will need to prepare a solution of certain strength from a given solution of another strength. Whenever solution preparation is required, accuracy is essential. When preparing a solution, it must be accomplished to exact specifications.

Preparing Solutions and Dilutions

Whenever a dilution is to be prepared, the formula is as follows:

Desired strength = X (amount needed)

Available strength amount available

Arterial Blood Gas Studies

Arterial blood gas studies (ABGs) are valuable tools in the treatment of critically ill patients. As the name suggests, ABGs are one of the few clinical laboratory procedures performed on arterial blood. Arterial blood gas analyzers quantitate ABG components using special electrodes. ABGs help assess a patient's ventilation, oxygenation, and acid-base balance. ABGs are also used to monitor the condition of critically ill patients, to diagnose electrolyte imbalances, to monitor oxygen flow rates, and to complement other pulmonary function studies. It should be remembered that any arterial puncture should not be attempted by anyone who is not trained and licensed to perform this procedure.

The Gram Stain

The Gram Stain is used to classify bacteria on the basis of their form, size, cellular morphology, and Gram Stain reaction. It is a critical test for the rapid presumptive identification of infectious agents, and it also is a means by which the quality of clinical specimen can be evaluated. When exposed to the Gram Stain, bacteria stain either gram-positive (deep violet) or gram-negative (light to dark red) on the basis of differences in cell wall composition and structure. Gram-positive bacteria have a thick peptidoglycan layer and large amounts of teichoic acids. This combination prevents them from being affected by alcohol decolorization; therefore, they retain the initial stain of crystal violet, which imparts a deep violet color. Gram-negative cell walls have a single peptidoglycan layer attached to a symmetric, lipoplysaccharide, phospholipid, bilayered, outer membrane interspersed with protein. The outer membrane is damaged by the alcohol decolorizer, allowing the crystal violet iodine complex to leak out and be replaced by the Sefranin counterstain (red). The Gram stain can be affected by many factors, including culturing, age, antibiotics, the medium in which the bacteria is growing, incubation, atmosphere, phagocytosis, and staining technique.

The most important bacterial property for classification purposes is a simple procedure that employs the aniline dye, crystal violet. The cell wall structure appears to be the determining factor by which bacteria react to the Gram stain.

Gram-positive bacteria: are bacteria that take up and retain the crystal violet and resist alcohol decoloration. They appear blue to black.

Gram-negative bacteria: are bacteria that are decolorized completely by ethanol and take up safranin counterstain. They appear red.

Gram staining is only a first step. Biochemical tests may have to be done before a final diagnosis is made. However, therapeutic decisions can be made based on this test.

The Gram staining procedure consists of the following sequence:

Dye – crystal violet

Mordant – Gram's iodine

Decolorizer – 95% ethyl alcohol/acetone mixture

Counterstain – safranin stain

Smear Preparation

Proper smear preparation will produce a thin monolayer of organisms for easy visualization but will be thick enough to reveal characteristic arrangements of the bacteria. Always wear latex gloves and a laboratory coat and follow all other universal precautions when handling clinical specimens.

Pre-cleaned, glass slides with frosted ends should be used for the smear. The frosted ends are desirable as they allow accurate labeling and convenient handling. Frequently, a direct smear is prepared from the swab used to obtain the sample. A smear can be from anybody opening, including the genitals or wounds (such as surgical sites, bites, cuts, or body ulcers). The best process is to obtain two swabs, one for the culture and one for the smear. If this is the case, the specimen is cultured first. Then, before the thioglycolate tube is inoculated, the smear is prepared. The danger in using one swab is that the target area may be missed, thus invalidating the entire testing process. You will want to check laboratory protocols for smear preparation to determine the exact procedure for obtaining a smear specimen.

Smearing and Fixation Technique

To prepare the smear, gently roll the swab across the slide, in one direction, leaving **a thin** film of specimen material on the slide. Specimens not received on swabs can be spread over a large area by using sterile swabs or a heat-sterilized wire loop to form a thin film on the slide. Extremely thick specimens can be placed on one slide, covered with a second slide, and pulled apart. The excess on the edge of the slide can be removed using a disinfectant-soaked paper towel. The smearing and fixation technique must be done in a bio safety cabinet.

Smears should be air-dried on a flat surface or on an electric slide warmer heated to 60 degrees Centigrade. The slide is placed on the supporting rods of the stain rack and then fixed by covering the slide with methanol for 1 minute. The residual methanol is then drained off without rinsing and is allowed to air-dry again. The slide is then ready to stain. Do no heat-fix the slide before staining. Methanol fixation is preferred over the old standard of heat-fixing smears because it prevents lysis of red blood cells (RBCs), gives a cleaner background, does not affect bacterial morphology, and is safer.

Staining Bacteria

The staining procedure involves the sequential application of primary stain mordant, decolorizer, and counterstain to a bacterial smear. The organisms according to the chemical composition of the cell walls take up the stains differently. A fixed smear is placed on a staining rack and the primary stain crystal violet is poured onto one end of the smear until the whole side is covered. The stain is allowed to remain in one place for 30 seconds.

Staining of Blood Smears

The stain commonly used for examination of blood cells is called polychromatic because they contain dyes that will stain various cell components different colors. These stains usually contain methylene blue, a blue stain, and eosin, a re-orange stain. These stains are attracted to different parts of the cell. Thus, the cells and their structures can be more easily visualized and differentiated. The most commonly used differential bloodstain is Wright's Stain. Semi-automated slide stainers are frequently used in large laboratories. These machines are capable of staining a large number of blood smears with consistency and reliability. Small laboratories generally use a manual quick stain method.

Urinalysis

Components of the urinary system

This system consists of two kidneys, two ureters, urinary bladder, and a urethra.

The kidney is the primary organ of the urinary system. The two kidneys are bean-shaped organs located on each side of the body behind the peritoneum on the back wall of the abdominal cavity. In cross-section, each kidney has an outer region, the renal cortex, and an inner region, the renal medulla. Urine flows from the collecting ducts to the renal pelvis and through the ureter into the bladder.

The kidneys' functions are: to remove metabolic waste from the blood stream, maintain the body's acid-base balance and regulate body hydration. Urea, a nitrogenous product of protein metabolism, is the major waste product removed by the kidney. The kidney's ability to reabsorb into the blood stream water and chemicals previously filtered from the blood allows it to regulate the acid-base and fluid balance of the body.

Hormones are also produced such as renin which controls blood pressure and erythropoietin which stimulates the production of red blood cells.

The two ureters are muscular tubes that carry urine from the kidney to the bladder. The bladder is an expandable sac located in the pelvis; it stores the urine formed by the filtration of blood in the glomerulus of the nephron. The urethra is the tube extending from the bladder to the external opening.

Anuria: The absence of urine

Hematuria: The presence of blood in urine

Polyuria: The passage of large volumes of urine

Proteinuria: The presence of excess proteins in urine

Collecting the Urine Specimen

The manner in which the specimen is collected depends on the test to be performed. In the medical office, the collection, processing, and/or transport of most specimens can be accomplished without complication. Patient education is the responsibility of the medical assistant, and collecting a urine specimen requires clear and concise instructions.

General Instructions for Urine Collection

Urine specimens may be collected in the medical office or at home. In either situation, it is important to follow appropriate procedures for specimen collection and processing.

Instructions for Urine Collection

1. Carefully label all specimens. Do not apply the label to the container lid, but place the label on the container itself. Use an indelible marker or make sure that the label will adhere to the container at refrigerated temperatures. On the label, record the patient's name, the date and time of collection, and the type of specimen. Add the physician's name if the specimen is to be sent to a central laboratory facility opening that is 2 inches in diameter. If the specimen is to be obtained from a pediatric patient, the container may be slightly smaller. If the specimen is to be transported, be sure it has a screw-type lid.

2. If a bacterial culture is ordered, make sure a sterile container is available. If this is the case, the specimen may have to be obtained through catheterization.

3. Advise female patients, with the consent of the physician, that the collection of a urine specimen should be avoided, if possible, during their menstrual cycle and for several days before and after, as the specimen may be contaminated with blood.

4. If the analyte is unstable or if the testing is delayed, you may add preservatives to the specimen. Check your laboratory's procedure manual or the procedural manual provided by the referral laboratory to determine the proper preservative for each test. Remember that the preservative must not interfere with the test procedure or results. Always note on the specimen the type and amount of preservative added.

Types of Specimen Collection

First Morning Sample

A first morning sample is the type of specimen most commonly used for routine urinalysis. Because the concentration of urine varies throughout the day, it is usually easiest to identify abnormalities in a relatively concentrated specimen. The first morning specimen may also be called an early morning specimen, as it represents the urine formed over approximately an 8-hour period.

Because it is impractical to collect a first morning specimen in the medical office, the patient must be instructed in the proper collection technique for a clean-catch or mid-stream urine sample. The specimen can then be collected at home and brought to the office. Be certain that the patient knows to refrigerate the specimen until it is transported to the office. The laboratory should supply the container, as a container from home may not be properly washed and rinsed prior to use. When the specimen is delivered to the office or laboratory, the medical assistant should check it for proper labeling and perform the required test(s) immediately. If that is not possible, the specimen may be refrigerated until testing can be done.

Mid-Stream Specimen

A mid-stream urine specimen is one that is collected not at the beginning or end of voiding, but in the middle of urination. The patient is instructed to void the first one third of the urine into the toilet. At the point, the patient stops urine flow, places the specimen container into position, and voids the next one third of the urine into the container. Once the specimen is collected, the patient can then finish emptying the bladder into the toilet. The specimen volume should be at least 25 mL of urine. A mid-stream specimen is thought to be a better representative of the contents of the bladder

Clean-Catch Specimen

Most laboratories prefer a clean-catch, mid-stream specimen for testing, as it provides the clearest, most accurate results. If the urine specimen is to be tested for bacteria or antibiotic sensitivity and a catheterized specimen is not required, a clean-catch sample will be needed. Collecting this sample requires special cleaning of the external genitalia. Because most patients are not familiar with aseptic technique, they must be carefully instructed on the procedure. In the case of a disabled or elderly individual, assistance may be needed in obtaining the specimen.

Urine composition

Urine formed by a healthy kidney is approximately 96% water and 4% dissolved substances consisting mainly of urea (a nitrogenous product of protein metabolism), sodium chloride, sulfates and phosphates. Abnormal constituents include RBCs and WBCs, fat, glucose, casts, bile, acetone, and hemoglobin. Other substances may be present in small quantities like calcium, hormones, proteins, fatty acids, and metals.

Urine Output

The actual amount of urinary output is dependent upon the body's state of hydration and normally averages 1200-1500ml every 24 hours. Decreased urinary output is termed oliguria. Increased output is called polyuria, and little or no urine output is known as anuria.

Routine Urinalysis

Examination of the urine is a diagnostic tool to detect or monitor certain conditions. It is often requested because urine is easily obtained and much information about the body can be had from the result of the test.

Examination of Urine

The routine urinalysis procedure is composed of three parts:

a. physical examination

b. chemical examination

c. microscopic examination

Physical examination of urine

This consists of:

i. Assessing the volume of the urine specimen to determine if it

ii. Is adequate for testing.

iii. Observing the color and appearance (or character) of the

iv. specimen

v. Noting the odor.

vi. Measuring the specific gravity.

Chemical examination of urine

This involves chemical evaluation of the contents of the urine which can be qualitative or quantitative. The chemical testing may involve examination of the following:

vii. pH

viii. Glucose

ix. Ketone

x. Protein

xi. Blood

xii. Bilirubin

xiii. Urobilinogen

xiv. Nitrite

xv. Leukocyte esterase

Microscopic examination of the urine

This is the microscopic examination done on urine sediment obtained by centrifugation of 10 to 15ml of urine. The identification and enumeration of the urinary sediment constituents require that only highly skilled and qualified individuals undertake the microscopic examination.

Specific Gravity

The specific gravity of urine is the ratio of the weight of a given volume of urine to the weight of the same volume of distilled water at a constant temperature. Specific gravity is the most convenient way of measuring the kidneys' ability to concentrate and dilute. An abnormality in the ability of the kidney to concentrate or dilute urine is an indication of renal disease or hormonal deficiency.

During a 24-hour period, normal adults with normal diets and normal fluid intake produce urine with a specific gravity of between 1.015 and 1.025. The normal range of urine specific gravity for a random collection is 1.005 to 1.030.

Urinary pH

The pH, or the percentage of hydrogen ion concentration of a solution, is a reflection of the acidity or alkaline of a solution. A pH of 7.0 is considered to be neutral. The pH of distilled water is 7.0. A pH of 0 to 7.0 is considered to be acidic, whereas a pH of 7 to 14 is considered to be alkaline or basic.

Normal, freshly voided urine will usually have a pH of 4.5 to 8.0. Within this range, the urine pH of most healthy patients is around 6.0.

Urinary Glucose

Glucose is the sugar typically found in urine. Other sugars, such as lactose, fructose, galactose, and pentose, may be detected in urine under specific circumstances. Glucose is present in urine when the blood glucose level exceeds the renal threshold. Glycosuria is the presence of glucose in the urine.

Patients with diabetes mellitus have glycosuria, along with polynuria and thirst. The reagent strip test for glucose relies on enzymatic tests that are specific for glucose. A common reagent strip urinary glucose enzymatic method uses glucose oxidase. The glucose oxidase reacts specifically with glucose. Sugars, such as lactose, fructose, and others, are not detected by the glucose oxidase method. A copper reaction test is a commonly used confirmatory and screening test for glucose and other reducing substances in urine. Copper reduction tests are used in pediatric patients to detect increased levels of glucose that may not be detected by the specific enzymatic test found on most reagent strips.

Urinary Bacteria

Enteric gram-negative bacteria that are always nitrite positive can convert urinary nitrate to nitrite. A positive nitrite test is an indication that a significant number of bacteria are present in the urine.

Urinary Leukocytes

The presence of increased numbers of leukocytes or white blood cells in the urine is an indicator of bacteriuria or urinary tract infection (UTI). Granulocytic leukocytes release esterase when the cells lyse. Testing for leukocyte esterase by the reagent strip method is used in tandem with the microscopic examination of urine sediment for the diagnosis of bacteriuria or UTI.

A positive test by the reagent strip method is indicated by a purple color. The greater the amount of leukocytes/esterase present, the greater the intensity of the purple color. Bacterial culture and sensitivity testing best confirm UTI's. A clean-catch mid-stream urine sample is usually required for any bacterial culture. For this reason, it is ALWAYS wise to collect a clean-catch urine specimen; do not dispose of the specimen until the physician directs you to do so.

Specialized Urine Tests/Urinary Pregnancy Testing

Probably the most common specialized urine test is the pregnancy test. Human chorionic gonadotropin (hCG), also known as uterine chorionic gonadotropin (UCG), is produced in the placenta and is detectable in the blood and urine early in the gestation period. HCG is not normally found in the urine of young, healthy, non-pregnant women. Because of hCG's early appearance during gestation, increased levels of hCG are a natural marker for pregnancy.

Other Specimen Collections

Hemoccult Fecal Occult Test

The Hemoccult Fecal Occult test is used to detect hidden blood in stool specimens. The first and last portion of the stool after the bowel movement usually contain concentrations of the substances most often required for testing. In order to conduct this test, a Hemmocult developing solution is applied to a stool specimen. Any trace of blue that appears within the specimen is a sign of a positive result.

Throat Culture

Throat cultures are used to detect a bacterial, fungal, or viral infection in the throat. In order to conduct this test, the patient should be placed in a comfortable lying or sitting position. After the patient has been asked to open their mouth, the medical assistant should depress the patient's tongue then vigorously swab the throat with a sterile swab. After the specimen is collected, it should be correctly labeled with the patient's information.

Sputum Specimen

A sputum specimen collection is used to determine the presence of pathogens in a patient's respiratory passage. When obtaining a sputum specimen, the medical assistant should instruct the patient to cough deeply, using the abdominal muscles as well as the accessory muscles to bring up secretions from the lungs as well as the upper airways. After the specimen is collected, it should be correctly labeled with the patient's information.

Legal Considerations

Informed consent

This is consent given by the patient who is made aware of any procedure to be performed, its risks, expected outcomes, and alternatives.

Patient confidentiality

This is the key concept of HIPAA. All patients have a right to privacy and all information should remain privileged. Discuss patient information only with the patient's physician or office personnel that need certain information to do their job. Obtain a signed consent form to release medical information to the insurance company or other individual.

Negligence

This is the failure to exercise the standard of care that a reasonable person would give under similar circumstances and someone suffers injury because of another's failure to live up to a required duty of care.

The four elements of negligence, (4 Ds), are:

1. Duty: duty of care

2. Derelict: breach of duty of care

3. Direct cause: legally recognizable injury occurs as a result of the breach of duty of care.

4. Damage: wrongful activity must have caused the injury or harm that occurred.

Tort

Is a wrongful act that results in injury to one person by another. Some examples of common torts that can occur in the clinic are the following:

1. *Battery* - The basis of tort in this case is the unprivileged touching of one person by another. When a procedure is to be performed on a patient, the patient must give consent in full knowledge of the procedure and the risk it entails (informed consent).

2. *Invasion of privacy* – This is the release of medical records without the patient's knowledge and permission.

3. *Defamation of character* – This consists of injury to another person's reputation, name, or character through spoken (slander) or written (libel) words.

Good Samaritan Law - This law deals with the rendering of first aid by health care professionals at the scene of an accident or sudden injury. It encourages health care professionals to provide medical care within the scope of their training without fear of being sued for negligence

Needle Stick Prevention Act

OSHA has put into force the Occupational Exposure to Bloodborne Pathogen (BBP) Standard when it was concluded that healthcare employees face a serious health risk as a result of occupational exposure to blood and other body fluids and tissues. The standards outline necessary engineering and work practice controls that OSHA believes will help minimize or eliminate exposure to employees. The standard was revised in 2001 to conform to the Needlestick Safety and Prevention Act passed in November 2000. The act directed OSHA to revise the BBP standard in four key areas:

- Revision and updating of the exposure control plan.

- Solicitation of employee input in selecting engineering and work practice controls.

-Modification of definitions relating to engineering controls (i.e., sharps disposal containers, self-sheathing needles, needleless systems.

- New record keeping requirements.

The employer must establish and maintain a sharps injury log for percutaneous injury from contaminated sharps and it must be done in such a manner to protect the confidentiality of the injured employee.

The sharps injury log must contain, at a minimum:

a. The type and brand of device involved in the incident.

b. The department or work area where the exposure incident occurred.

c. An explanation of how the incident occurred.

AN OVERVIEW OF ANATOMY AND PHYSIOLOGY OF THE HUMAN BODY

In this section, the entire body will be studied. The various body systems, organs, tissues, and positional and directional terms will be addressed.

Organs

Organs are comprised of several types of tissue. The stomach is made up of muscle tissue, nerve tissue, and epithelial tissue. The medical term for internal organs is viscera.

Systems are groups of organs working together to perform complex functions.

Body Systems Functions Organs

Musculoskeletal support, movement muscles, bones, joints, bone protection marrow

Integumentary: protection skin, hair, nails

Gastrointestinal: nutrition stomach, intestines

Urinary: elimination of nitrogenous kidneys, bladder, ureters, waste urethra

Reproductive: reproduction ovaries, testes

Blood/Lymphatic: transportation blood cells

Immune: protection

Cardiovascular: transportation lymph glands heart, vessels

Respiratory: delivers oxygen to cells lungs, bronchi, trachea removes carbon dioxide

Nervous/Behavioral: receive/process information brain, nerves, mind

Endocrine: effects changes through pancreas, thyroid

Body Cavities

The body is divided into five cavities. Two of these cavities are in the back of the body and are called **dorsal** cavities. The positional term is **posterior**. The other three cavities are in the front of the body and are called **ventral** cavities. The positional term is called **anterior**. The cranial cavity and the spinal cavity are the two dorsal cavities. The ventral cavities are the thoracic cavity which is divided into two smaller cavities; the **pleural** and the **mediastinum**. The pleural cavity is the space surrounding each lung, and the **mediastinum** contains the heart, aorta, trachea, etc. The diaphragm, a muscle, separates the thoracic cavity from the abdominal cavity. The abdominal cavity contains the stomach, the small and large intestines, spleen, pancreas, liver
and gallbladder. The pelvic cavity contains the rectum, urinary bladder, urethra and ureters; uterus and vagina in the female. Due to the fact that there is nothing that separates the abdominal cavity and the pelvic cavity, they are often referred to as the abdominopelvic cavity.

Planes of the Body

Dividing the body into planes or flat surfaces is an additional way to describe the body. These descriptions listed below are useful when doing magnetic imaging, CT scans, and other imaging techniques.

Sagittal planes are vertical planes that separate the sides from each other.

Midsagittal plane separates the body into right and left halves.

The **frontal plane** divides the body into front and back portions.

The **transverse plane** divides the body horizontally into an upper and lower part.

Positional and Directional Terms

Anterior (ventral) – front surface of the body

Posterior (dorsal) – back side of the body

Deep – away from the surface

Proximal –near the point of attachment to the trunk or near the beginning of a structure.

Distal – far from the point of attachment to the trunk or far from the beginning of a structure.

Inferior – below another structure

Superior – above another structure

Medial – pertaining to the middle or nearer the medial plane of the body

Lateral – pertaining to the side

Supine – lying on the back

Prone – lying on the belly

Musculoskeletal System

The musculoskeletal system includes the bones, muscles, and joints. The bones are connected to one another by fibrous bands of tissue called **ligaments**. Muscles are attached to the bone by tendons. The fibrous covering of the muscles is called the fascia and the articular cartilage covers the end of many bones and serves as a protective function. The musculoskeletal system acts as a framework for the organs, protects many of those organs, and also provides the organism the ability to move.

Bones

Bones are complete organs made up of connective tissue called **osseous**. The inner core of bones is comprised of **hematopoietic** tissue. This is where the red bone marrow manufactures blood cells. Other parts of the bone are storage areas for minerals necessary for growth. Examples of these minerals are calcium and phosphorous.

Types of bones

Bones are categorized as belonging to either the **axial skeleton** or the **appendicular skeleton**. The axial skeleton consists of the skull, rib cage, and spine. The appendicular skeleton is made up of the shoulder, collar, pelvic and arms and legs.

Bones come in a variety of shapes and sizes. The following is a description of shapes of human bones and where they are located.

Long bones are typically very strong, are broad at the ends and have large surfaces for muscle attachment. The humerus and the femur are large bones. **Short bones** are small with irregular shapes. They are found in the wrist and ankle. **Flat bones** are found covering soft body parts. These are the shoulder blades, ribs, and pelvic bones. **Sesamoid bones** are small, rounded bones that resemble a sesame seed. They are found near joints and increase the efficiency of muscles near a joint. An example of sesamoid bone is the patella.

Bone Landmarks

Crest- Ridge of bone

Spine-sharp, narrow projection

Condyle-knuckle shaped portion of bone

Process- projection of bone

Tubercle- small, rounded projection

Tuberosity- a projection

Foramen-a rounded orifice in the bone

Sinus-cavity inside of bone

Sulcus- a groove in the bone

Joints

Synarthrosis-an immovable joint

Amphiarthrosis- a slightly movable joint

Diathrosis-a freely movable joint

The Axial Skeleton – Skull, Spine, Rib Cage

The skull is made up of two parts, the cranium and the facial bones. The cranium includes the following bones:

Frontal Bone – forms the anterior part of the skull and the forehead

Parietal Bones – forms the sides of the cranium

Occipital Bone – forms the back of the skull. There is a large hole at the ventral surface in this bone, called the foramen magnum, which allows the brain communication with the spinal cord.

Temporal Bone – forms the two lower sides of the cranium.

Ethmoid Bone – forms the roof of the nasal cavity.

Sphenoid Bones – anterior to the temporal bones.

Facial Bones

Zygoma – Cheekbone

Lacrimal bones – paired bones at the corner of each eye that cradle the tear ducts.

Maxilla – upper jaw bone

Mandible – lower jaw bone

Vomer – bone that forms posterior/inferior part of the nasal septal wall between the nostrils.

Palatine bones – make up part of the roof of the mouth

Inferior nasal conchae – make up part of the interior of the nose.

Spinal/Vertebral Column

The spinal / vertebral column is divided into five regions from the neck to the tailbone. There are 26 bones in the spine and they are referred to as the **vertebrae.** The following list explains the bones of the spine:

Cervical Neck Bones

Thoracic Upper back

Lumbar Lower back

Sacral Sacrum

Coccygeal Coccyx (tailbone)

Rib Cage

There are 12 pairs of ribs. The first 7 pairs join the sternum anteriorly through cartilaginous attachments called costal cartilages. The **true ribs**, numbers 1-7, attach directly to the sternum in the front of the body. **False ribs**, numbers 8-10, are attached to the sternum by cartilage. Ribs 11 and 12 are **floating ribs**, because they are not attached at all.

The Appendicular Skeleton

The **upper appendicular** skeleton includes the shoulder girdle which is made up of the **scapula, clavicle and upper extremities**. The **scapula**, or shoulder blades are flat bones that help support the arms. The **clavicle**, or collarbone, is curved horizontal bones that attach to the upper sternum at one end. These bones help stabilize the shoulder. The **upper extremities** consist of the following:

The **humerus** which is the upper arm bone.

The **ulna** is the lower medial arm bone.

The **radius** is the lateral lower arm bone (in line with the thumb).

The **carpals** are wrist bones. There are 2 rows of four bones in the wrist.

The **metacarpals** are the five radiating bones in the fingers. These are the bones in the palm of the hand.

The **phalanges** (phalanx.s) are the finger bones. Each finger has three phalanges, except for the thumb. The three phalanges are the proximal, middle and a distal phalanx. The thumb has a proximal and distal.

Lower Appendicular

The lower half of the appendicular skeleton can be divided into the pelvis and the lower extremities.

Pelvis: superior and widest bone

Ischium: lower portion of the pelvic bone

Pubic bone: the lower anterior part of the bone

Lower Extremities

Femur: thighbone

Patella: kneecap

Tibia: shin

Fibula: smaller, lateral leg bone

Malleolus: ankle

Tarsal: hind foot bone

Metatarsal: midfoot bone

Phalanx: toe bones, 14 in all (2 in the great toe, 3 in each of the other toes)

Fractures

A fracture is a broken bone. Most fractures occur as a result of trauma, however some diseases like cancer or osteoporosis can also cause spontaneous fractures. Fractures can be classified as simple or compound. Simple fractures do not rupture the skin, as compound fractures split open the skin allowing for an infection to occur. Compound fractures are considered an emergent situation.

Types of Fractures

Comminuted – the bone is crushed and or shattered.

Compression – the fractured area of bone collapses on itself.

Colles – the break of the distal end of the radius at the epiphysis often occurs when the patient has attempted to break his or her fall.

Complicated – the bone is broken and pierces an internal organ

Impacted – the bone is broken and the ends are driven into each other.

Hairline – A minor fracture appears as a thin line on x-ray and may not extend completely through the bone.

Greenstick – the bone is partially bent and partially broken; this is a common fracture in children because their bones are still soft.

Pathologic – any fracture occurring spontaneously as a result of disease.

Salter-Harris – a fracture of the epiphyseal plate in children.

Muscles

Muscle is tissue composed of cells. Muscles have the ability to contract and relax. The muscles in the human body have three different functions: 1. to allow the skeleton to move, 2. Responsible for movement of organs, and 3. to pump blood to the circulatory system. Muscles are attached to bones by strong, fibrous bands of connective tissue called tendons.

Muscle Actions

Action Description

Extension: to increase the angle of a joint

Flexion: to decrease the angle of a joint

Abduction: movement away from the midline

Adduction: movement towards the midline

Supination: turning the palm or foot upward

Pronation: turning the palm or foot downward

Dorsiflexion: raising the foot, pulling the toes toward theshin

Plantar flexion: lowering the foot, pointing the toes away from the shin

Eversion: turning outward

Inversion: turning inward

Protraction moving: a part of the body forward

Retraction moving: a part of the body backward

Rotation: revolving a bone around its axis

Sprains, strains and dislocation/subluxation

A **sprain** is a traumatic injury to a joint involving the soft tissue. The soft tissue includes, the muscles, ligaments, and tendons. A strain is a lesser injury, usually this is a result of overuse or overstretching. Dislocation is when a bone is completely out of place and subluxation is partially out of joint.

The Integumentary System

The skin and its accessory organs make up the **integumentary** system. Integument means covering. The skin covers over an area of 22 square feet (an average adult). It is a complex system of specialized tissues containing glands, nerves and blood vessels. The main function of the skin is to protect the deeper tissues from excessive loss of minerals, heat, and water. It also provides protects the body from diseases by providing a barrier. The skin is the largest organ of the body and accomplishes its diverse functions with assistance from the hair, nails, and glands. The **sebaceous(oil) glands** and the **suddoriferous (sweat) glands** produce secretions that allow the body to be moisturized or cooled. Nerve fibers help the body adjust to the environment by sensory messages relayed to the brain and spinal cord. Other tissues in the skin maintain body temperature. Nerve fibers also help blood vessels to dilate and sweat gland to produce sweat. There are three layers to the skin: the **epidermis**, the **dermis**, and the **subcutaneous layer**. The epidermis is a thin, cellular membrane layer that contains keratin. The dermis is a dense, fibrous, connective tissue that contains collagen. The subcutaneous layer is a thicker and fatter tissue.

Hair, Nails and Glands

Hair fibers are composed of tightly fused meshwork of cells filled with hard protein called **keratin.** The hair has its roots in the dermis and together with their coverings, is called hair follicles. The main function of the hair is to assist in the regulation of body temperature. It holds heat in when the body is cold by standing on end and holding a layer of air as insulation. Nails cover and protect the dorsal surfaces of the distal bones of the fingers and toes. The part that is visible is the nail body, the nail root is under skin at the base of the nail and the nail bed is the vascular tissue under the nail that appears pink when the blood is oxygenated or blue/purple

when it is oxygen deficient. The moon like white area at the base of the nail is called the **lunula**. There is also the cuticle at the lower part of the nail and this is sometimes referred to as the **eponychium.**

Sebaceous glands are located in the dermal layer of the skin over the entire body, except for the palms of the hands and soles of the feet. The sebaceous glands secrete an oily substance called **sebum**. Sebum contains lipids that help lubricate the skin and minimize water loss. It is the overproduction of sebum during puberty that contributes to acne in some people.

Sweat glands are tiny, coiled gland found on almost all body surfaces. They are most numerous in the palms and soles of the feet. Coiled sweat glands originate in the dermis and straighten out to extend up through the epidermis. The tiny opening on the surface is a **pore.** There are two types of sweat glands: **eccrine sweat glands** are the most common and the **apocrine sweat glands** that secrete an odorless sweat.

ANATOMY OF THE EYE

There are outer protective layers of the eye known as the sclera), cornea, ciliary body, choroid, and the iris. The sclera is the white outer part of the eye which covers the front of the eye. The cornea covers the front of the eyeball, and deflects light rays as they enter the eye. The choroid prevents the reflection of light within the eyeball. The ligaments of the ciliary body contains the vitreous-humor, a transparent, colorless fills the eyeball in front of the retina. The iris is the colored part of the eye.

ANATOMY OF THE EAR

The ear is divided into three regions which are known as the external ear, the middle ear, and the inner ear. The external region encompasses the outer surface of the tympanic membrane along with the auricle (pinna), external auditory meatis, and the external auditory canal. The middle ear is inclusive of the tympanic membrane and the middle ear cleft. Other structures within this region are the ossicles, along the opening of both the eustachian and the mastoid cavity.

The inner ear contains structures such as the bony labyrinth, cochlea, endolymph, and the semicircular canals.

ANATOMY OF THE NOSE

The outer portion of the nose is none as the external meatus, the triangular shaped projection located in the center of the face. The two chambers of the nose are known as the external nostrils.

These chambers are divide by the septum which consists of bone and cartilage. Other structures of the nose include the nasal passages and the sinuses.

ANATOMY OF THE NECK

The neck is divided into two large triangles that are separated by the sternocleidomastoid muscle.

The triangle located closer to the upper portion of the body is known as the submandibublar triangle. This region contains the submandiublar gland as well as the hypoglossal nerve. The lower triangle is known as the cervical triangle which is traversed by the digastric muscle. Other structures of the neck include the carotid arteries, internal jugular vein, the larynx, pharynx, and the thyroid gland.

ANATOMY OF THE SHOULDER

The two main bones of the shoulder are the humerus and the scapula. Four short muscles originate on the scapula and pass around the shoulder where their tendons fuse together to form the rotator cuff:

Supraspinatus

Infraspinatus

Teres minor

Subscapularis

The end of the scapula, which is known as the genoid, meets the head of the humerus to form a glenohumeral cavity that acts as a flexible ball-and-socket joint.

Section 2

Contents in this section

Introduction

Anatomy & Physiology : An overview of the skin and the heart

Site Selection

Venipuncture

Complications associated with phlebotomy

Factors to consider prior to carrying out the procedure

Quality assurance and specimen handling

Analytical errors

Routine venipuncture

Failure to obtain blood

Special venipuncture

Special specimen handling

Dermal Punctures/Micro Capillary collection

Order of draw

Test tubes, additives and tests

Safety

Infection control/ chain of infection

Legal considerations in phlebotomy

References

Practice test One

Practice Test Two

Clinical Laboratory Sections

The clinical laboratories have various sections and these subdivisions are made depending on the size and specialties within such laboratories. Various laboratory sections perform special tests as categorized within their expertise. For instance, the Hematology department is responsible for the tests of the formed or cellular elements of blood such as red blood cells, platelets and white blood cells. Both quantitative and qualitative tests are carried out in the department such as number and size or shape or maturity (Lindh, Poole, Tamparo, & Dahl, 2010). The blood components' ability to perform their individual tasks correctly is also tested in the hematology department.

The parasitology section is where ova and parasite tests are performed on specimens while microscopic examination of cells are performed to detect early signs of cancer and other diseases is carried in the cytology section. Frozen samples of biopsies are sliced, stained and then examined microscopically for cancer and other diseases in the histology section. (Lindh, Poole, Tamparo, & Dahl, 2010)

Hematology Section

This is the section where the formed elements of the blood are studied by enumerating and classifying the red blood cells, white blood cells, and platelets. By studying and examining the cells, disorders and infections are detected and treatment instituted or monitored. Whole blood is the most common specimen analyzed and usually collected in lavender-top tube containing the anti-coagulant EDTA.

Aside from complete blood count (CBC), which is the primary analysis performed, other tests such as: Erythrocyte sedimentation rate (ESR), Lupus erythematosus (LE) prep, Reticulocyte (retic) count, and Sickle cell. The coagulation section is usually a part of hematology. However, in large laboratories they are separated. This is the area where hemostasis is evaluated. Plasma is usually the specimen analyzed, drawn from blood collected in light-blue top tube with the anticoagulant sodium citrate. The tube must be inverted three to four times. Some of the tests frequently performed in the coagulation area are: Activated partial thromboplastin time (APTT); Thrombin Time (TT); Prothrombin time (PT); Bleeding Time (BT).

Chemistry Section

The most automated section in the laboratory. This section is divided into several areas:

☐ **Electrophoresis** – analyzes chemical components of blood such as hemoglobin and serum, urine and cerebrospinal fluid, based on the differences in electrical charge.

☐ **Toxicology** - analyzes plasma levels of drugs and poisons.

☐ **Immunochemistry** – This section uses techniques such as radio immunoassay (RIA) and enzyme immunoassay to detect and measure substances such as hormones, enzymes, and drugs.

Some tests in the chemistry section are ordered by profiles, which are groups of tests ordered by a physician to evaluate the status of an organ, body system or general health of the patient. Examples of these profiles are:

☐ Liver profile: tests may include ALP, AST, ALT, GGT and Bilirubin

☐ Coronary risk profile: tests may include Cholesterol, Triglycerides, HDL, LDL

Blood Bank Section

This is the section where blood is collected, stored and prepared for transfusion. Strict adherence to procedures for patient identification and specimen handling is a must to ensure patient safety. Blood collected may be separated into components: packed cells, platelets, fresh frozen plasma, and cryoprecipitate.

Serology (Immunology) Section

Performs tests to evaluate the patient's immune response through the production of antibodies. This section uses serum to analyze presence of antibodies to bacteria, viruses, fungi, parasites and antibodies against the body's own substances (autoimmunity).

Microbiology Section

This section is responsible for the detection of pathogenic microorganisms in patient samples and for the hospital infection control. The primary test performed is culture and sensitivity (C&S). It is used to detect and identify microorganisms and to determine the most effective antibiotic therapy. Results are usually available within 24 to 48 hours; but cultures for tuberculosis and fungi require several weeks. One instance when culture and sensitivity is used is to diagnose the cause of a patient's fever of unknown origin (FUO).

Urinalysis Section

This section performs tests on the urine to detect disorders and infection of the kidney and urinary tract and to detect metabolic disorders such as diabetes mellitus. Urinalysis has three components:

☐ Physical examination- evaluates the color, clarity and specific gravity

☐ Chemical examination- determines pH, glucose, ketones, protein, blood, bilirubin, urobilinogen, nitrites, and leukocytes.

☐ Microscopic examination- identifies presence of casts, bacteria, yeast, and parasites.

Anatomy and Physiology: An Overview of the Circulatory System and the Skin

A phlebotomist should understand the blood circulatory system and the composition of blood so as to be able to collect blood from an individual or patient. For instance, blood forms in the body organs, and the bone marrow is responsible for the formation of blood cells. Blood is produced in sites such as the spleen, thymus and the lymph nodes (Lindh, Poole, Tamparo, & Dahl, 2010). Blood performs crucial functions in the body such as transporting oxygen to body tissues and organs and removing carbon dioxide from such organs and tissues, the waste product of functions of the organs and tissues. In addition, blood carries nutrients to all parts of the body and removes wastes products, which it moves to organs such as the kidney, lungs, liver and the skin for excretion (Lindh, Poole, Tamparo, & Dahl, 2010).

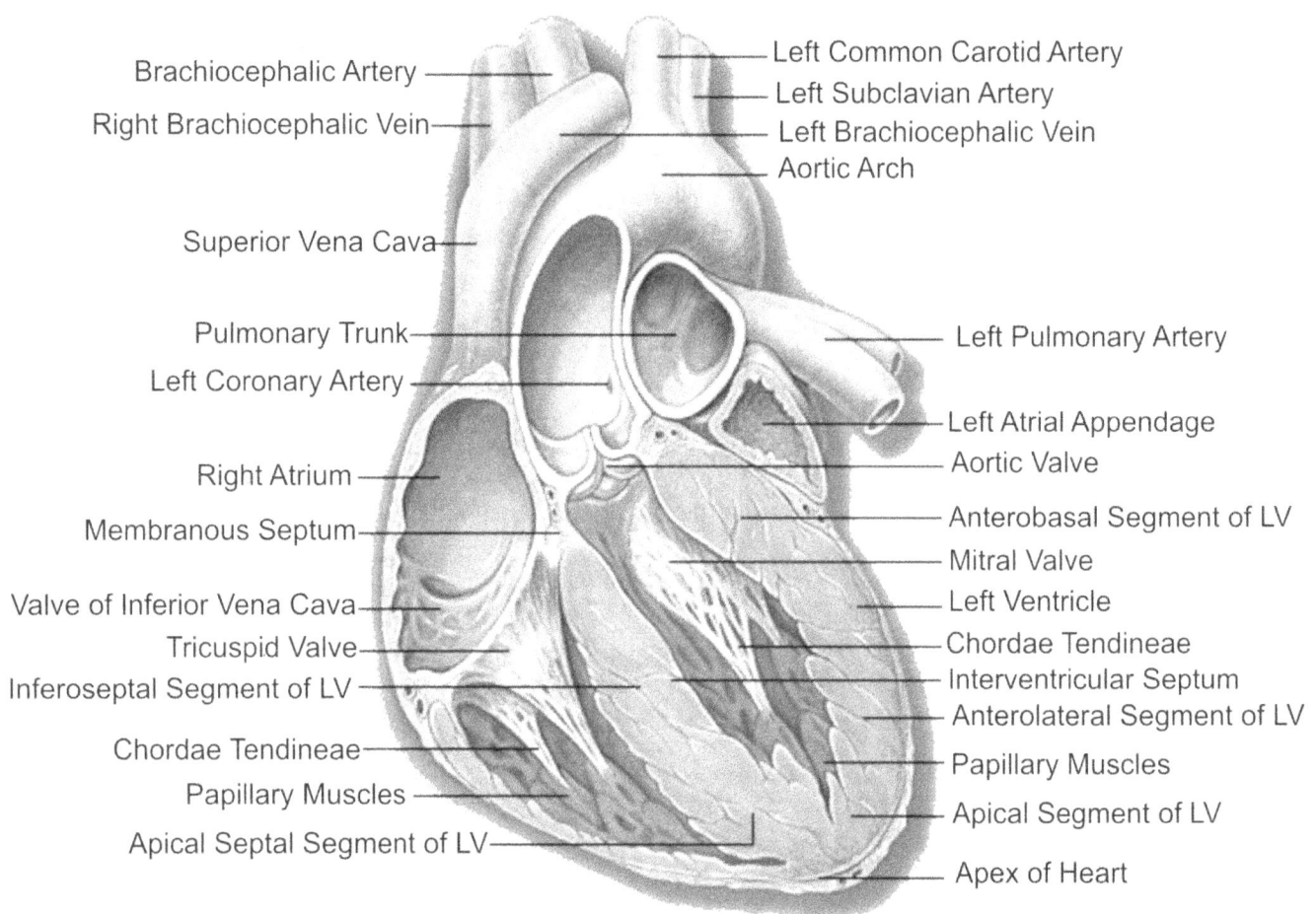

Brachiocephalic Artery — Left Common Carotid Artery
Right Brachiocephalic Vein — Left Subclavian Artery
— Left Brachiocephalic Vein
— Aortic Arch
Superior Vena Cava —
Pulmonary Trunk — — Left Pulmonary Artery
Left Coronary Artery — — Left Atrial Appendage
— Aortic Valve
Right Atrium — — Anterobasal Segment of LV
Membranous Septum — — Mitral Valve
— Left Ventricle
Valve of Inferior Vena Cava — — Chordae Tendineae
Tricuspid Valve — — Interventricular Septum
Inferoseptal Segment of LV — — Anterolateral Segment of LV
Chordae Tendineae — — Papillary Muscles
Papillary Muscles — — Apical Segment of LV
Apical Septal Segment of LV — — Apex of Heart

Components of the blood circulatory system include the heart, veins, arteries and capillaries. The heart is responsible for the pumping of blood through the body in arteries, veins and capillaries (Lindh, Poole, Tamparo, & Dahl, 2010). Arteries enable blood to flow away from the heart while blood flows into the heart through veins. Capillaries connect veins and arteries. Arteries are thick walled to enable them withstand pressure, and they normally branch to form arterioles which also branch to form capillaries (Lindh, Poole, Tamparo, & Dahl, 2010). Capillaries join to form venules which supply blood back to the veins. Blood is composed of the liquid part which is plasma, red blood cells, platelets and white blood cells (Hoeltke, 2013).

The circulatory system is divided into two systems: the pulmonary system and the systemic system. Blood is circulated to the lungs for enrichment with oxygen and removal of carbon dioxide through the pulmonary system while the systemic system supplies cells with oxygen, fats carbohydrates and other energy sources, as well as, removes waste products (Hoeltke, 2013). The skin is made of three layers.

These are the epidermis, the dermis and the hypodermis from the outermost to the innermost respectively.

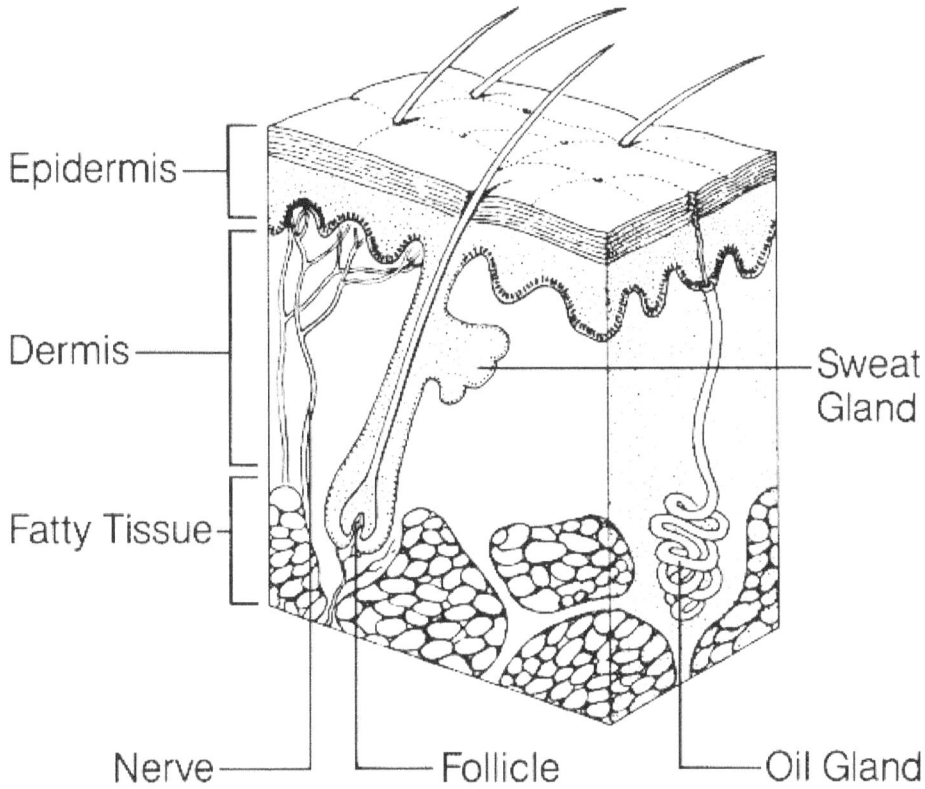

The circulatory system

The function of this system is to deliver oxygen, nutrients, hormones, and enzymes to the cells (exchange is done at the capillary level) and to transport cellular waste such as carbon dioxide and urea to the organs (lung and kidneys, respectively) where they can be expelled from the body. It is a transport system where the blood is the vehicle; the blood vessels, the tubes, and the heart work togethernwith the heart working as a pump.

The heart

The heart acts as two pumps in series (right and left sides), connected by two circulations, with each pump equipped with two valves, the function of which is to maintain a one-way flow of blood. The two circulations are:

1. Pulmonary circulation - this carries deoxygenated blood from the right ventricle to the lungs (oxygenation takes place at the alveoli) and returns oxygenated blood from the

lungs to the left atrium.

2. Systemic circulation – this carries oxygenated blood from the left ventricle throughout the body.

Each side of the heart (right and left) is composed of an upper chamber, the atrium, and a lower chamber, the ventricle. The right side has two valves:

The tricuspid valve – this is an atrioventricular valve, being situated between the right atrium and right ventricle.

The pulmonic valve – a semi lunar valve situated between the right ventricle and the pulmonary artery.

The left side also has two valves: The mitral valve (also known as the bicuspid valve) – this is another atrioventricular valve, being situated between the left atrium, and left ventricle.

The aortic valve – a semi lunar valve situated between the left ventricle and the aorta.

The heart has three layers:

Endocardium - The endothelial inner layer lining of the heart.

Myocardium - The muscular middle layer. This is the contractile element of the heart.

Epicardium - The fibrous outer layer of the heart. The coronary arteries, which supply blood to the heart, are found in this layer.

The blood vessels

The blood vessels are: Aorta, arteries, arterioles, capillaries, venules, veins, superior and inferior vena cavae.

The blood vessels, except for the capillaries, are composed of three layers. The outer connective tissue layer is called the tunica adventitia. The middle smooth muscle layer is called the tunica media. The inner endothelial layer is called the tunica intima.

The aorta, arteries, and arterioles carry oxygenated blood from the heart to the various parts of the body; while the venules, veins and the superior and inferior vena cavae carry deoxygenated blood back to the heart.

The capillaries, composed only of a layer of endothelial cells, connect the arterioles and venules. As such, capillary blood is a mixture of arterial and venous blood. The thin walls allow rapid exchange of oxygen, carbon dioxide, nutrients and waste products between the blood and tissue cells.

Blood

The average adult has 5 to 6 liters of blood. It is composed of a liquid portion called the 'plasma', and a cellular portion called the 'formed elements'. Plasma comprises 55% of the circulating blood and it contains proteins, amino acids, gases, electrolytes, sugars, hormones, minerals, vitamins, and water (92%). It also contains waste products such as urea that are destined for excretion.

The formed elements constitute the remaining 45% of the blood. They are **erythrocytes** (red blood cells), which comprise 99% of the formed elements, the leukocytes (white blood cells) and the **thrombocytes** (platelets). All blood cells normally originate from stem cells in the bone marrow.

The **erythrocytes** contain hemoglobin, the oxygen-carrying protein. It enters the blood as an immature reticulocyte where in one to two days, it matures into an erythrocyte. There are 4.2 to 6.2 million RBC's (red blood cells) per microliter of blood. The normal life span of an RBC is 120 days.

The **leukocytes** function is to provide the body protection against infection. The normal amount of WBC's (white blood cells) for an adult is 5,000 to 10,000 per microliter. Leukocytosis, which is an increase in WBCs, is seen in cases of infection and leukemia. Leukopenia, which is a decrease in WBCs, is seen with viral infection or chemotherapy.

There are five types of WBCs in the blood. A differential count determines the percentage of each type:

Neutrophils – the most numerous, comprise about 40% to 60% of WBC population. They are phagocytic cells, meaning, they engulf and digest bacteria. Their number increases in bacterial infection, and often, the first one on the scene.

Lymphocytes - the second most numerous, comprising about 20% to 40% of the WBC population. Their number increases in viral infection, and they play a role in immunity.

Monocytes – comprising 3% to 8% of the population, they are also the largest WBCs. They are monocytes while in the circulating blood, but when they pass into the tissues, they transform into macrophages and become powerful phagocytes. Their number increases in intracellular infections and tuberculosis.

Eosinophils - represent 1% to 3% of the WBC population. They are active against antibody-labeled foreign molecules. Their numbers are increased in allergies, skin infections, and parasitic infections.

Basophils - account for 0% to 1% of WBCs in the blood. They carry histamine, which is released in allergic reactions

The **thrombocytes** (platelets) are small irregularly shaped packets of cytoplasm formed in the bone marrow from megakaryocytes. Essential for blood coagulation, the average number of platelets is 140,000 to 440,000 per micro liter of blood. They have a life span of 9 to 12 days.

HEMOSTASIS

Hemostasis is the process by which blood vessels are repaired after injury. This process starts from vascular contraction as an initial reaction to injury, then to clot formation, and finally removal of the clot when the repair to injury is done. It occurs in four stages:

Stage 1: Vascular phase

Injury to a blood vessel causes it to constrict slowing the flow of blood.

Stage 2 – Platelet phase

Injury to the endothelial lining causes platelets to adhere to it.

Additional platelets stick to the site finally forming a temporary platelet plug in a process called 'aggregation'. Vascular phase and platelet phase comprise the primary hemostasis. Bleeding time test is used to evaluate primary hemostasis.

Stage 3 – Coagulation phase

This involves a cascade of interactions of coagulation factors that converts the temporary platelet plug to a stable fibrin clot. The coagulation cascade involves an intrinsic system and extrinsic system, which ultimately come together in a common pathway.

Activated partial thromboplastin time (APTT) – test used to evaluate the intrinsic pathway. This is also used to monitor heparin therapy.

Prothrombin time (PT) – test used to evaluate the extrinsic pathway. This is also used to monitor coumadin therapy.

Stage 4 – Fibrinolysis

This is the breakdown and removal of the clot. As tissue repair starts, plasmin (an enzyme) starts breaking down the fibrin in the clot. Fibrin degradation products (FDPs) measurement is used to monitor the rate of fibrinolysis.

Site Selection

The appropriate venipuncture site varies, depending on the patient. The bend of the upper arm should be checked first, normally called the antecubital area. Here, the median cubital vein is the primary and prominent vein that should be looked for, and is normally found in the middle bend of the arm. Alternatively, a phlebotomist can use basilic, cephalic or median veins as alternative choices (Hoeltke, 2013). A phlebotomist should choose a site that will give the best blood return such as the ankle or foot, wrist, in line with the thumb, back of the hand, upper arm, and antecubital area.He/she should avoid sites such as Edematous arms, arms in casts, cannulas, fistulas, arm with intravenous fusion, areas of scarring and the side of a mastectomy.

A tourniquet will help fill the veins with blood by constricting the flow of blood and it should be placed three to four inches above the proposed site. Look for a vein by feeling with the tip of an index finger or middle finger because these fingers are more sensitive than the thumb which has a pulse (Hoeltke, 2013). Palpate and trace the path of the vein several times. The roundness and direction of the vein should be identified because not all veins go straight up or down the arm. In case the vein that has been identified pulsates, then that is not a vein but an artery and it should not be punctured. Avoid probing (sideways needle manouvers) during venipunctures to avoid tampering with nerves.

The preferred site for venipuncture is the antecubital fossa of the upper extremities. The vein should be large enough to receive the shaft of the needle, and it should be visible or palpable after tourniquet placement.

Three major veins are located in the antecubital fossa, and they are:

A. **Median cubital vein** – the vein of choice because it is large and does not tend to move when the needle is inserted.

B. **Cephalic vein** - the second choice. It is usually more difficult to locate and has a tendency to move, however, it is often the only vein that can be palpated in the obese patient.

C. **Basilic vein** - the third choice. It is the least firmly anchored and located near the brachial artery. If the needle is inserted too deep, this artery may be punctured.

Unsuitable veins for venipuncture are:

A. **Sclerosed veins** - These veins feel hard or cordlike. Can be caused by disease, inflammation, chemotherapy or repeated venipunctures.

B. **Thrombotic veins**

C. **Tortuous veins** – These are winding or crooked veins. These veins are susceptible to infection, and since blood flow is impaired, the specimen collected may produce erroneous test results.

Note: Do not draw blood from an arm with IV fluids running into it. The fluid will alter the test results. Select another site. If the patient has IVs on both arms, ask the RN to turn off the IV for 30 minutes, then draw. Do not draw blood from an artificial a-v fistula site, such as those surgically implanted in dialysis patients.

Venipuncture

Venipuncture involves a procedure of puncturing into a vein to obtain blood samples. Healthcare professionals normally use three methods to perform venipuncture: the vacuum tube method, the butterfly method and the syringe method (Lindh, Poole, Tamparo, & Dahl, 2010). Phlebotomists should have options when they are required to draw blood from a variety of patients in different situations. In all the methods used to perform venipuncture, the blood is transferred to a vacuum tube, be properly selected and used while there should be proper labeling procedures and which contains the chemicals and substances that are necessary for blood tests to be carried out (Lindh, Poole, Tamparo, & Dahl, 2010). The basic step in performing venipuncture is to have the necessary supplies and/or equipment organized for proper collection of specimen and to ensure the patient's safety and comfort. The recommended supplies are as follows:

A. Laboratory requisition slip and pen.

B. Antiseptic –

☐ Prepackaged 70% isopropyl alcohol pads are the most commonly used.

☐ For collections that require more stringent infection control such as blood cultures and arterial punctures Povidone-iodine solution is commonly used.

☐ For patients allergic to iodine, chlorhexidine gluconate is used.

C. Vacutainer tubes –

☐ Color-coded for specific tests and available in adult and pediatric sizes.

D. Vacutainer needles-

☐ These are disposable and are used only once both for single-tube draw and multidraw (more than one tube).

☐ Needle sizes differ both in length and gauge. 1-inch and 1.5-inch long are routinely used.

☐ The diameter of the bore of the needle is referred to as the gauge. The smaller the gauge the bigger the diameter of the needle; the bigger the gauge the smaller the diameter of the needle (i.e. 16 gauge is large bore and 23 gauge is small bore.) Needles smaller than 23 gauge are not used for drawing blood because they can cause hemolysis.

E. Needle adapters -

☐ Also called the tube holder. One end has a small opening that connects the needle, and the other end has a wide opening to hold the collection tube.

F. Winged infusion sets -

☐ Used for venipuncture on small veins such as those in the hand. They are also used for venipuncture in the elderly and pediatric patients.

☐ The most common size is 23gauge, ½ to ¾ inch long.

G. Sterile syringes and needles -

☐ 10-20 ml syringe is used when the Vacutainer method cannot be used.

H. Tourniquets –

☐ Prevents the venous outflow of blood from the arm causing the veins to bulge thereby making it easier to locate the veins.

☐ The most common tourniquet used is the latex strip. (Be sure to check for latex allergy). Tourniquets with Velcro and buckle closures are also available.

☐ Blood pressure cuffs may also be used as tourniquet. The cuff is inflated to a pressure above the diastolic but below the systolic.

I. Chux –

☐ An impermeable pad used to protect the patient's clothing and bedding.

J. Specimen labels -

☐ To be placed on each tube collected after the venipuncture.

K. Gloves -

☐ Must always be worn when collecting blood specimen

L. Needle disposal container –

☐ Must be a clearly marked puncture-resistant biohazard disposal container.

☐ **Never recap a needle without a safety device.**

Complications Associated with Phlebotomy

Sometimes, healthcare professionals experience problems in obtaining a blood specimen. This occurs when a blood sample cannot be obtained. Probing should not be attempted because as the needle is moved sideways, it slices the patient's tissues, thereby causing avoidable injury. A secondvenipuncture may be performed, but a venipuncture should not be attempted more than twice. Other complications may arise such as hematoma, which forms under the skin adjacent to the puncture site (Medtexx Medical Corporation, 2007). Petechiae form little, red spots, consisting of extravasated blood as a result of a coagulation abnormality such as platelet defect. Phlebotomy is also associated with fainting (syncopy) of patients when they think of blood or when they see it, just because their blood was drawn (Medtexx Medical Corporation, 2007). It is helpful to ask the patient if they have fainting spells when their blood is drawn. If they answer in the affirmative, make sure they sit down for 30 minutes after the venipuncture to avoid syncope.

☐ **Hematoma:** The most common complication of phlebotomy procedure. This indicates that blood has accumulated in the tissue surrounding the vein. The two most common causes are the needle going through the vein, and/or failure to apply enough pressure on the site after needle withdrawal.

☐ **Hemoconcentration:** The increase in proportion of formed elements to plasma caused by the tourniquet being left on too long. (More than two (2) minutes)

☐ **Phlebitis:** Inflammation of a vein as a result of repeated venipuncture on that vein.

☐ **Petechiae:** These are tiny non-raised red spots that appear on the skin from rupturing of the capillaries due to the tourniquet being left on too long or too tight.

☐ **Thrombus:** This is a blood clot usually a consequence of insufficient pressure applied after the withdrawal of the needle.

☐ **Thrombophlebitis:** Inflammation of a vein with formation of a clot

☐ **Septicemia:** This is a systemic infection associated with the presence of pathogenic

organism introduced during a venipuncture.

☐ **Trauma:** This is an injury to underlying tissues caused by probing of the needle.

Factors to Consider Prior to Performing the Procedure

Prior to performing phlebotomy, it should be ensured that the patient is properly identified using correct

procedures. Equipment should be ready and laboratory requisitions should be visible (Medtexx Medical

Corporation, 2007). Phlebotomists should consider the order of draw in cases of multiple tube specimens.

In addition, phlebotomists should identify the venipuncture sites and ensure safety of the patient (Medtexx

Medical Corporation, 2007).

☐ **Fasting** – some tests such as those for glucose, cholesterol, and triglycerides require that the patient

abstain from eating for at least 12 hours. The phlebotomist must ascertain that the patient is indeed in a

fasting state prior to the testing.

☐ **Edema** –is the accumulation of fluid in the tissues. Collection from edematous tissue

alters test results.

☐ **Fistula -** is the permanent surgical connection between an artery and a vein. Fistulas are used for

dialysis procedures and must never be used for venipunctures due to the possibility of infection.

Quality Assurance and Specimen Handling

There should be proper handling of specimen beginning the time blood is drawn into the evacuated tube or

syringe and during the collection process, as well as transportation and processing of the specimen in the

laboratory. Specimens should be handled with utmost concern for blood-borne pathogen safety to protect

the healthcare professional and others from potentially infectious substances (Kalanick, 2004). Needles

and sharps should be monitored to ensure that they are sterile before use. Tubes and other equipment must be used and disposed appropriately (Ridley, 2011). Also, specimens should be properly labeled and protected from lighting.

Quality assurance (QA) is defined as a program that guarantees quality patient care by tracking the outcomes through scheduled audits in which areas of the hospital look at the appropriateness, applicability, and timeliness of patient care. A QA program is a continuous program, established by the healthcare facility, which will provide guidelines, protocols and continuing education for their employees. Areas in phlebotomy that are subject to quality control:

Patient preparation procedures:

Quality control actually starts before the specimen is collected from the patient. To obtain an acceptable specimen, the patient must be prepared properly. In a hospital setting the phlebotomist must check the records' book, to ensure that the nursing department has performed all pre-test preparations. Pre-test preparation will include fasting for specific tests. The phlebotomist must then ensure this information is correct, by asking the patient. The Laboratory/Phlebotomy Specimen Collection Procedures Manual has established these guidelines.

Analytical Errors

Analytical errors occur during the process of analysis or testing of the specimens in phlebotomy. Venipuncture sites should be chosen properly because they may be a potential source of analytical errors and risk to the patient (Prince, 2011). These errors are caused by issues such as poor faulty instrumentation and lack of highly skilled testing personnel. Also, the way the specimen is handled and stored may alter the results obtained through testing.

Before Collection	During Collection	After Collection.
Patient misidentification	Extended tourniquet time	Failure to separate serum from cell
Improper Time of Collection	Hemolysis	Improper use of serum separator
Wrong Tube	Wrong order of draw	Processing delays

Inadequate fast   Failure to invert tubes   Exposure to light

Exercise   Faulty technique   Improper storage conditions

Patient posture   Under filling tubes   Rimming clots

Poor coordination with other treatments

Improper site preparation

Medication interference

Routine Venipuncture

Blood should be collected from the antecubital, the median cubital and the cephalic veins, which should be punctured using the evacuated collection system or the syringe or butterfly collection system, in an aseptic manner (Davis B. K., 2010). A phlebotomist should not insert a needle above an intravenous infusion site. Phlebotomists should allow outpatients to sit for fifteen minutes to let the body to recover from stress before attempting a venipuncture. He/she should release the tourniquet and remove the needle, immediately they discover the venipuncture has begun swelling during the venipuncture process (Kalanick, 2004).

1) Verify the requisition for the tests.

2) Identify the patient: check the patient's ID number and have him/her state his/her name.

3) Identify yourself to the patient, explain the procedure, and secure his/her consent.

4) Palpate the veins in the antecubital fossa using your index finger.

5) Gather the necessary equipment.

6) Wash hands; put on gloves.

7) Tie on the tourniquet; it should be applied 3-4 inches above the site where the venipuncture will be made. Ask the patient to make a fist or open and close his/her hand to help engorge the vein.

8) Palpate the vein while looking for the straightest point. Cleanse the area using a circular

motion starting at the inside of the venipuncture site.

9) Assemble the needle and tube holder while the alcohol is drying. Uncap the needle and examine it for defects such as blunted or barbed point.

10) Hold the patient's arm, by placing four fingers under the forearm and your thumb below the antecubital area slightly pulling the skin back to anchor the vein.

11) With the bevel facing upward, insert the needle at an angle of 15-30 degrees.

12) Once the needle is inside the vein (you will feel a "give" as the vein is entered), push the collection tube into the holder to puncture the tube stopper with the back-end of the needle.

13) Release the tourniquet once blood flow has begun. The tourniquet should not be left on for more than one (1) minute in order to prevent hemoconcentration.

14) Fill the needed tubes, according to the order of draw.

15) Pull out collection tube from the holder.

16) Place folded gauze over the venipuncture site and withdraw the needle. Then apply pressure until bleeding stops. This is done to prevent hematoma. Do not ask the patient to bend the arm as it does not offer enough pressure.

17) Discard needle into the biohazards sharp container.

18) Label each collected specimen, writing the patient's name and ID number, the time and date of collection, and your initials.

19) Place labeled tubes inside the biohazards transport bag.

20) Before leaving, check the venipuncture site. If it is still bleeding, apply pressure for another 2 minutes. If after this time, it is still bleeding, continue to apply pressure for another 3 minutes. If bleeding persists after a total of 8 minutes of applying pressure, call for help.

21) At any point when the bleeding stops, an adhesive bandage is applied over a folded gauze square. The patient should be instructed to remove the bandage within an hour.

22) Clean up everything and dispose of waste properly.

23) Leave the patient's call light within his/her reach.

24) Remove the gloves, wash your hands, say good-bye to the patient and inform him/her that his/her physician will deliver the results.

☐ Do not label the tubes prior to the venipuncture.

☐ Do not leave the patient's room before labeling the tubes.

☐ Do not dismiss an outpatient before labeling the tubes.

☐ Do not label tubes using a pencil; black ink should be used.

☐ Do not leave the patient until you checked and ensure that the bleeding has stopped.

Failure to obtain Blood

Failure to obtain blood is termed as failed venipuncture. When this occurs, a phlebotomist needs to change the position of the needle by rotating it half a turn. A failed venipuncture may result when the bevel of the needle is against the wall of the vein, indicating that the needle has not penetrated the vein far enough (Hoeltke, 2013). In this case, the phlebotomist is required to advance the needle a little bit further, but to be careful not to go too deep. This is because only a small change makes the difference between a failed and a successful venipuncture. Alternatively, when the needle has been pushed too far into the vein, a phlebotomist may fail to obtain blood and he or she needs to pull the needle back a little. The needle should be pulled back slowly when there is an unsuccessful venipuncture, and the blood will start coming almost immediately as it seems the needle is ready to come out of the skin (Hoeltke, 2013).

There are other reasons for failed venipuncture. For instance, the tube may have pulled back out of the holder. Sometimes, the tubes do not stay pushed all the way into the holder while the blood is being collected, and may slide back out leading to a stoppage in filling with blood. The ideal remedy in this situation is to exert slight pressure on the tube into the holder (Hoeltke, 2013). Also, the tube that is in use for drawing blood may not have sufficient vacuum. This requires a phlebotomist to try another tube before withdrawing. Most venipunctures are routine, but in some instances, complications can arise resulting in failure to obtain blood. The following are some of the common causes:

☐ The tube has lost its vacuum. This is may be due to:

o A manufacturing defect

o Expired tube

o A very fine crack in the tube

☐ Improperly positioned needle. In many instances, slight movement of the needle can correct this.

o The bevel of the needle is resting against the wall of the vein. Slightly rotate the needle.

o The needle is not fully in the vein. Slowly advance the needle.

o The needle has passed through the vein. Slowly pull back on the vein.

o The vein was missed completely. With a gloved finger, gently determine the positions of the vein and the needle, and redirect the needle.

☐ Collapsed vein. This may be due to excessive pull from the vacuum tube; use of a smaller vacuum tube may remedy the situation. If it does not, remove the tourniquet, withdraw the needle, and select another vein preferably using either a syringe or butterfly.

Another reason for failing to obtain blood is when the tourniquet is too tight, stopping blood flow. To remedy the problem, the tourniquet should be reapplied loosely. The arm can be massaged and the venipuncture location can be warmed. Finally, a phlebotomist may use a blood pressure cuff, inflated to between the patient's systolic and diastolic pressure. This provides a larger service area to apply pressure, which can be regulated to bring veins to the surface when other methods have failed (Hoeltke, 2013).

<h1 style="text-align:center">Special Venipuncture</h1>

Special venipuncture results when it is difficult to draw blood from a patient using routine venipuncture. This is normally associated with Edema of the extremities, scarring or burn patients, post mastectomy patients and dialysis patients. Therefore venipuncture should not be performed in Edematous areas, scarring or burnt areas, and fistula or on the same side of the mastectomy (Turgeon, 2005). Some venipunctures are done using special collecting or handling procedures specific to the test being requested. Some require patient preparation such as fasting, while some needs to be collected at a specific time. Still, others may need special handling such as protection from light.

Fasting Specimens

This requires collection of blood while the patient is in the basal state, that is, the patient has fasted and refrained from strenuous exercise for 12 hours prior to the drawing. It is the phlebotomists responsibility to verify if the patient indeed, has been fasting for the required time.

Timed Specimens

They are often used to monitor the level of a specific substance or condition in the patient. Blood is drawn at specific times for different reasons. They are:

- To measure blood levels of substances exhibiting diurnal variation. (e.g., cortisol hormone)

- To determine blood levels of medications. (e.g., digoxin for cardiovascular disease)

- To monitor changes in a patient's condition. (e.g., steady decrease in hemoglobin level)

Two-Hour Postprandial Test

This test is used to evaluate diabetes mellitus. Fasting glucose level is compared with the level 2 hours after eating a full meal or ingesting a measured amount of glucose.

Oral Glucose Tolerance Test (OGTT)

This test is used to diagnose diabetes mellitus and evaluate patients with frequent low blood sugar. 3-hour OGTT is used to test hyperglycemia (abnormally high blood sugar level) and diagnose diabetes mellitus. 5-hour OGTT is used to evaluate hypoglycemia (abnormally low blood sugar level) for disorders of carbohydrate metabolism. OGTT are scheduled to begin between 0700 and 0900.

Therapeutic Drug Monitoring

This test is used to monitor the blood levels of certain medication to ensure patient safety and also maintain a plasma level. Blood is drawn to coincide with the trough (lowest blood level) or the peak level (highest blood level). Trough levels are collected 30 minutes before the scheduled dose. Time for collecting peak level will vary depending on the medication, patient's metabolism, and the route of administration (I.V., I.M., or oral).

Blood Cultures (BC)

They are ordered to detect presence of microorganisms in the patient's blood. The patient will usually have chills and fever of unknown origin (FUO), indicating the possible presence of pathogenic microorganisms in the blood (septicemia). Blood cultures are usually ordered STAT or as timed specimen, and collection requires strict aseptic technique.

PKU

This test is ordered for infants to detect phenylketonuria, a genetic disease that causes mental retardation and brain damage. Test is done on blood from newborn's heel or on urine.

SPECIAL SPECIMEN HANDLING

Cold Agglutinins

Cold agglutinins are antibodies produced in response to Mycoplasma pneumoniae infection (atypical pneumonia). The antibodies formed may attach to red blood cells at temperatures below body temperature, and as such, the specimen must be kept warm until the serum is separated from the cells. Blood is collected in red-topped tubes pre-warmed in the incubator at 37 degrees Celsius for 30 minutes.

Chilled specimens

Some tests require that the specimen collected be chilled immediately after collection in crushed ice or ice and water mixture. Likewise, the specimen must be immediately transported to the laboratory for processing. Some of the tests that require chilled specimen are: arterial blood gases, ammonia, lactic acid, pyruvate, ACTH, gastrin, and parathyroid hormone.

Light-sensitive specimens

Specimens are protected from light by wrapping the tubes in aluminum foil immediately after they are drawn. Exposure to light could alter the test results for: Bilirubin, beta-carotene, Vitamins A & B6, and porphyrins.

DERMAL PUNCTURES (Microcapillary collection)

When venipuncture is inadvisable, it is possible to perform a majority of laboratory tests on micro samples obtained by dermal (skin) puncture, with the exception of ESR, blood cultures and other tests that require a large amount of serum. Dermal puncture may be done on both pediatric and adult patients.

Punctures should never be performed with a surgical blade or hypodermic needle because they can be difficult to control. Deep penetration into the skin can cause serious injury such as osteomyelitis (inflammation of the bone and bone marrow). A lancet should be used, which delivers a pre-determined depth that can range from 0.85mm for infants to 3.0 mm for adults.

Site selection for dermal puncture

Infants:

The heel is used for dermal punctures on infants less than 1 year of age. Areas recommended are the medial and lateral areas of the plantar surface of the foot. These are determined by drawing imaginary lines medially extending from the middle of the great toe to the heel and laterally from the middle of the fourth and fifth toes to the heel.

The American Academy of Pediatrics recommends that heel punctures for infants not exceed 2.0mm.

Observe the following precautions when performing dermal puncture:

☐ do not puncture deeper than 2.0mm

☐ do not perform dermal punctures on previous puncture sites

☐ do not use the back of the heel or arch of the foot.

☐ use the medial and lateral areas of the plantar surface of the heel

Older children and Adults

The distal segment of the third or fourth finger of the non-dominant hand is the recommended site. Puncture is made in the fleshy portion of the finger slightly to the side of the center perpendicular to the lines of the fingerprint.

Dermal puncture procedure

1. Identify the patient

2. Assemble equipment

3. Warm the site: this is an essential part of the procedure when collecting specimens for pH or blood gases. Warming the site can increase the blood flow up to seven times the normal amount. The specimen is referred to as arterialized specimen because of the increase arterial flow to the area. This is accomplished by warming the site for a minimum of three minutes with a warm moistened towel (no greater than 108 F), or with a commercial warming device.

4. Clean the site: Use 70% isopropyl alcohol. Allow the site to dry for maximum antiseptic action. Alcohol residue can cause hemolysis of the red blood cells and may interfere with glucose testing. Povidone- iodine (Betadine) is not used for cleaning the site because it interferes with several tests like bilirubin, uric acid, phosphorous, and potassium.

5. Prepare the puncture device

6. Perform the dermal puncture

Order of draw for capillary specimens

1. Lavender tube

2. Tubes with other additives

3. Tubes without additives

Microsamples are labeled with the same information required for venipuncture specimens.

Special Specimen Handling

During phlebotomy, there are specimens which require special handling after collection. These are specimens that have special requirements. Such specimens include those that should be protected from light, those that need to be chilled and those that need to be kept warm (McCall & Tankersley, 2003). Therefore, phlebotomists should ensure that they handle special specimens appropriately for accuracy of the test results for patients. Dermal Punctures/Micro Capillary Collection. Phlebotomists perform the venipuncture procedure most frequently. However, this procedure is not appropriate in all circumstances. Laboratory test can be performed on micro samples of blood that are obtained by dermal puncture on adult and pediatric patients as a result of advances in laboratory instrumentation and the need for point of care testing (Strasinger & Lorenzo, 2011). Dermal puncture is performed on the skin or capillaries, and is normally used to collect blood from infants and children who are below two years of age. This is because it is difficult to locate superficial veins that are large enough to be penetrated by even a small gauge needle in infants and children below two years, and available veins need to be reserved for intravenous therapy.

Use of deep veins may be dangerous and cause complications such as cardiac arrest among such patients. In addition, if excessive amounts of blood are drawn from infants can lead to anemia (Strasinger & Lorenzo, 2011). Finally, capillary blood is required in certain tests such as newborn screening tests and capillary blood gases. In adults, dermal puncture is performed on burnt or scared patients, patients receiving chemotherapy and patients with thrombotic tendencies. Also patients with fragile veins, inaccessible veins, as well as, obese and apprehensive patients are ideal for dermal puncture (Strasinger & Lorenzo, 2011).

Order of Draw

Normally, most of the blood collection tubes contain an additive which either facilitates or prevents the specimen from clotting. At times, additive carry-over from one tube to the next can occur, altering results drastically. Additive carry-over occurs when blood or anticoagulant mixture is transferred by the needle used to fill one tube into the next tube filled (Ernst, 2005). This can lead to wrong diagnosis, which is dangerous because it prevents physician intervention.

Wrong order of draw may lead to cross-contamination of anticoagulants and contaminate blood culture collections. Since the tops of blood collection tubes are not sterile, the needles that puncture them are likely to pick up and transport bacteria from one tube to the next (Ernst, 2005). If the next tube is a blood culture bottle the culture could be contaminated and lead the laboratory to report a positive blood culture on a patient who does not have bacterial blood infection. This may lead to wastage of funds and prolonged stay in hospital for unnecessary medication and tests.

Therefore, it is recommended that blood cultures should be collected before other tubes are filled. The order of draw has significant impacts on patient results and physicians' responses to the results. Therefore, the following order should be followed. The tubes for blood cultures should come first, followed by tubes containing sodium citrate. These are followed by serum tubes with or without clot activators or gel separators and then tubes containing heparin. Tubes containing EDTA follow and finally, tubes containing sodium fluoride (Davis, 2002). Often requests are for more than one test to be performed; and as such, more than one collection

tube needs to be drawn. The correct order of draw is:

First — blood culture tubes or vials;

Second — sodium citrate tubes (e.g., blue tops);

Third — serum tubes with or without clot activator or gel; (e.g., red tops);

Fourth — heparin tubes (e.g., green tops);

Fifth — EDTA tubes (e.g., lavender tops);

Sixth — oxalate/fluoride tubes (e.g., gray tops).

Test Tubes, Additives and Tests

The correct tube or specimen container should be used. This means that phlebotomists must follow the manufacturer's instructions, pertaining to tubes and additives to ensure accurate test results and that no microclots form in the tubes. There should be proper checking of all tubes for cracks and expiry dates.

Additives should be observed whether they have discoloration, which could indicate contamination while new lot numbers of tubes must be checked to verify draw and fill accuracy (Rodak, 2007). Test tubes are used to collect blood specimen and normally packed with rubber stoppers (DeLaune & Ladner, 2010). They also contain specific substances or chemicals for tests to be run. It is important to read the label to determine the additive that is in the tube when a phlebotomist is in doubt (Gibson, Shah, & Umberger, 2013).

Safety

There should be safety provisions which should be followed for the safety of the patient and that of the phlebotomy technician. Safety must be followed so as to prevent the patient from contracting an infection. Similarly, the healthcare professional should not be vulnerable to acquiring a disease from patients while working. New needles and clean gloves should be used always. Medical assistants, phlebotomists and nurses should try to avoid the use of needles as much as possible, if other effective alternatives are available. Devices with safety features should be used always (Hoeltke, 2013). Priorities and strategies for prevention should be authorized by examination of local and national risk factors information. Proper training of health workers should be instituted to enhance safe use and disposal of needles and sharps (Hoeltke, 2013).

Infection Control/Chain of Infection

Infections can be contracted through different methods. Therefore, there should be proper washing of hands and phlebotomists should adhere to universal precautions strictly. There should be isolation of body substance and identification of patients who are at risk for susceptibility, treating their underlying conditions where possible and isolating them. Medical asepsis should be observed (Lindh, Poole,

Tamparo, & Dahl, 2010). Medical asepsis aims at destroying pathologic organisms so as to decrease the risk for transmission to others. Therefore, it should be ensured that objects are medically aseptic when such objects are to be used in (Lindh, Poole, Tamparo, & Dahl, 2010).

Infection Control/Chain Of Infection

This consists of links, each of which is necessary for the infectious disease to spread. Infection control is based on the fact that the transmission of infectious diseases will be prevented or stopped when any level in the chain is broken or interrupted.

Agent ------------- Mode of transmission ------------ Susceptible host

      portal of exit : :   portal of entry: :

Agents– are infectious microorganisms that can be classified into groups namely: viruses, bacteria, fungi, and parasites. When infectious diseases are identified according to the specific disease-causing microorganism, the disease may be prevented with the use of anti-infective drugs or infection control practices.

Portal of exit –the method by which an infectious agent leaves its reservoir. Standard Precautions and Transmission-Based Precautions are control measures aimed at preventing the spread of the disease as infectious agents exit the reservoir.

Mode of transmission –specific ways in which microorganisms travel from the reservoir to the susceptible host. There are five main types of mode of transmission:

- Contact : direct and indirect

- Droplet

- Airborne

- Common vehicle

- Vectorborne

Portal of entry – allows the infectious agent access to the susceptible host. Common entry sites are broken skin, mucous membranes, and body systems exposed to the external environment such as the respiratory, gastrointestinal, and reproductive. Methods such as sterile wound care, transmission-based precautions, and aseptic technique limit the transmission of the infectious agents.

Susceptible host – The infectious agent enters a person who is not resistant or immune. Control at this level is directed towards the identification of the patients at risk, treat their underlying condition for susceptibility, or isolate them from the reservoir.

Medical Asepsis

Best defined as "the destruction of pathogenic microorganisms after they leave the body." It also involves environmental hygiene measures such as equipment cleaning and disinfection procedures. Methods of medical asepsis are Standard Precautions and Transmission-Based Precautions.

Handwashing

Hand washing is the most important means of preventing the spread of infection. A routine hand wash procedure uses plain soap to remove soil and transient bacterial. Hand antisepsis requires the use of antimicrobial soap to remove, kill or inhibit transient microorganisms. It is important that all healthcare personnel learn proper hand washing procedures.

Barrier Protection

Protective clothing provides a barrier against infection. Used properly, it will provide protection to the person wearing it; disposed of properly it will assist in the spread of infection. Learning how to put on and remove protective clothing is vital to insure the health and wellness of the person wearing the PPE. PPE's or personal protective equipment includes:

☐ Gloves – worn for three reasons:

☐ Gloves are worn to provide protective barrier and to prevent gross contamination of the hands when touching blood, body fluids, secretions, excretions, mucous membranes, and nonintact skin.

☐ Gloves are worn to reduce the likelihood that microorganisms present on the hands of personnel will be transmitted to patients during invasive or other patient-care procedures that involve touching a patient's mucous membranes and nonintact skin.

☐ Gloves are worn to reduce the likelihood that hands of personnel contaminated with microorganisms from a patient or a fomite can transmit these microorganisms to another patient.

☐ Masks

☐ Goggles

☐ Face Shields

☐ Respirator

Isolation Precautions

For many years, the CDC recommended universal precautions, which is a method of infection control that assumed that all human blood and blody fluids were potentially infectious. The CDC issued a revised guidelines consisting of two tiers or levels of precautions: Standard Precautions and Transmission-Based Precautions.

Standard Precautions

This is an infection control method designed to prevent direct contact with blood and other body fluids and tissues by using barrier protection and work control practices.

Under the standard precautions, all patients are presumed to be infective for blood-borne pathogens. Infection control practices to be used with all patients. These replace universal precautions and body substance isolation. They are used when there is a possibility of contact with any of the following:

☐ Blood

☐ All body fluids, secretions, and excretions (except sweat), regardless of whether

or not they contain visible blood

☐ Nonintact skin

☐ Mucous membranes designed to reduce the risk of transmission of microorganisms from both

☐ Recognized and unrecognized sources of infections.

The standard precautions are:

☐ Wear gloves when collecting and handling blood, body fluids, or tissue specimen.

☐ Wear face shields when there is a danger for splashing on mucous membranes.

☐ Dispose of all needles and sharp objects in puncture-proof containers without recapping.

Transmission- Based Precautions the second tier of precautions and are to be used when the patient is known or suspected of being infected with contagious disease. They are to be used in addition to standard precautions. All types of isolation are condensed into three categories:

Contact precautions: are designed to reduce the risk of transmission of microorganisms by direct or indirect contact. Direct-contact transmission involves skin-to-skin contact and physical transfer of microorganisms to a susceptible host from an infected or colonized person. Indirect-contact transmission involves contact with a contaminated intermediate object in the patient's environment

Airborne precautions: are designed to reduce the risk of airborne transmission of infectious agents. Microorganisms carried in this manner can be dispersed widely by air currents and may become inhaled by or deposited on a susceptible host within the same room or over a longer distance from the source patient. Special air handling and ventilation are required to prevent airborne transmission.

Droplet precautions: are designed to reduce the risk of droplet transmission of infectious agents. Droplet transmission involves contact with the conjunctivae or the mucous membranes of the nose or mouth of a susceptible person with large particle droplets generated from the source person primarily during coughing, sneezing, or talking. Because droplets generally travel only short distances, usually three feet or less, and do not remain suspended in the air, special air handling and ventilation are not required. Safety hazards abound in the healthcare setting, many of which can cause serious injury or disease. The Occupational Safety and Health Administration (OSHA) is responsible for the identification of the various hazards present in the workplace and for the creation of rules and regulations to minimize exposure to such hazards. Employers are mandated to institute measures that will assure safe working conditions and health workers have the obligation to know and follow those measures.

Types of Hazards

☐ **Biologic**: infectious agents that can cause bacterial, viral, fungal, or parasitic infections.

☐ **Sharps**: needles, lancets, and broken glass can puncture and cut and cause bloodborne pathogen exposure.

☐ **Chemical**: preservatives and chemicals used in the laboratory. There is possible exposure to toxic, carcinogenic or caustic substances.

☐ **Electrical:** high-voltage equipment can cause burns and shock.

☐ **Fire or explosive**: Bunsen burners, oxygen and chemicals can cause burns or dismemberment.

☐ **Physical**: wet floors, heavy lifting can cause falls, sprains and strains.

☐ **Allergic reaction**: latex sensitivity that can cause allergic reactions ranging from simple dermatitis to anaphylaxis.

Emergency First Aid

The ability to recognize and react quickly to an emergency may be the difference of life or death for the patient. As patients react differently to various situations, it is important for all healthcare professionals to be prepared in an emergency.

External Hemorrhage: controlling the bleeding is most effectively accomplished by elevating the affected part above heart level and applying direct pressure to the wound. Do not attempt to elevate a broken extremity as this could cause further damage.

Shock occurs when there is 'insufficient return of blood flow to the heart, resulting in inadequate supply of oxygen to all organs and tissues of the body.' Patients experiencing trauma may go into shock and for some patients, seeing their own blood may induce shock. Common symptoms:

☐ Pale, cold, clammy skin

☐ Rapid, weak pulse

☐ Increased, shallow breathing rate

☐ Expressionless face/staring eyes.

First Aid for Shock:

☐ Maintain an open airway for the victim

☐ Call for assistance

☐ Keep the victim lying down with the head lower than the rest of the body

☐ Attempt to control bleeding or cause of shock (if known)

☐ Keep the victim warm until help arrives

Cardiopulmonary Resuscitation. Most healthcare institutions require their professionals to be certified in CPR. It is important for all professionals to maintain all certifications acquired.

Disinfection. the third procedure used in medical asepsis using various chemicals that can be used to destroy many pathogenic microorganisms. Since chemicals can irritate skin and mucous membranes, they are used only on inanimate objects.

The least expensive and most readily available disinfectant for surfaces such as countertops is a 1:10 solution of household bleach. Boiling water (temperature of 212 F) is considered a form of disinfection, but use of it in today's medical setting is limited to items that:

1. will not be used in invasive procedures;

2. will not be inserted into body orifices nor be used in a sterile procedure.

Latex Sensitivity

Latex sensitivity is an emerging and important problem in the health care field. Following the development of Universal Precaution Standards (OSHA, 1980), the use of natural rubber latex gloves for infection control skyrocketed. Within the last decade, however, the incidence of latex sensitivity has grown. Every health care worker must be concerned about latex sensitivity. Individuals with a known sensitivity to latex should wear a medical alert bracelet.

Legal Considerations in Phlebotomy

Phlebotomists should not violate the legal rights of patients because this may lead to legal action. Therefore, phlebotomists should consider the rights of patients to be professionally binding. Confidentiality is among the principal legal issues in phlebotomy. This encourages intimate level communication between phlebotomists and a patient. Confidentiality prohibits phlebotomists from disclosing some information that they gain to third parties without the consent of the original source of such information (Davis B. K., 2010). In turn, this will exclude unauthorized people from getting access to client information. Phlebotomists should practice confidentiality because clients may fail to disclose personal information which may be vital for their care and treatment. Phlebotomists' self discipline when dealing with patient information is crucial.

Another legal issue is legal refusal of treatment by patients. For instance, it is common for phlebotomists to face situations in which a patient refuses to have blood drawn. Phlebotomists are expected to respect such a decision (Davis B. K., 2010). This means that phlebotomists should not attempt to proceed and perform phlebotomy to avoid legal suits for patient battery, which is intentionally touching another person without authorization to do so. Instead, proper explanations should be provided to the refusing patients that it is the doctor who has ordered the tests and that the doctor needs the test results for making treatment decisions. Where patients insist and continue refusing, phlebotomists should notify appropriate people such as physicians and nurses and document the client's refusal (Davis, 2002).

Needle Stick Prevention Act

OSHA has put into force the Occupational Exposure to Bloodborne Pathogen (BBP) Standard when it was concluded that healthcare employees face a serious health risk as a result of occupational exposure to blood and other body fluids and tissues. The standards outline necessary engineering and work practice controls that OSHA believes will help minimize or eliminate exposure to employees. The standard was revised in 2001 to conform to the

Needlestick Safety and Prevention Act passed in November 2000. The act directed OSHA to revise the BBP standard in four key areas:

- Revision and updating of the exposure control plan.

- Solicitation of employee input in selecting engineering and work practice controls.

- Modification of definitions relating to engineering controls (i.e., sharps disposal containers, self-sheathing needles, needleless systems.

- New record keeping requirements.

The employer must establish and maintain a sharps injury log for percutaneous injury from contaminated sharps and it must be done in such a manner to protect the confidentiality of the injured employee.

The sharps injury log must contain, at a minimum:

a. The type and brand of device involved in the incident.

b. The department or work area where the exposure incident occurred.

c. An explanation of how the incident occurred.

Informed consent

This is consent given by the patient who is made aware of any procedure to be performed, its risks, expected outcomes, and alternatives.

Patient confidentiality

This is the key concept of HIPAA. All patients have a right to privacy and all information should remain privileged. Discuss patient information only with the patient's physician or office personnel that need certain information to do their job. Obtain a signed consent form to release medical information to the insurance company or other individual.

Negligence

This is the failure to exercise the standard of care that a reasonable person would give under similar circumstances and someone suffers injury because of another's failure to live up to a required duty of care. The four elements of negligence, (4 Ds), are:

1. Duty: duty of care

2. Derelict: breach of duty of care

3. Direct cause: legally recognizable injury occurs as a result of the breach of duty of care.

4. Damage: wrongful activity must have caused the injury or harm that occurred.

Tort

Is a wrongful act that results in injury to one person by another. Some examples of common torts that can occur in the clinic are the following:

Battery - The basis of tort in this case is the unprivileged touching of one person by another. When a procedure is to be performed on a patient, the patient must give consent in full knowledge of the procedure and the risk it entails (informed consent).

Invasion of privacy – This is the release of medical records without the patient's knowledge and permission.

Defamation of character – This consists of injury to another person's reputation, name, or character through spoken (slander) or written (libel) words.

Good Samaritan Law - This law deals with the rendering of first aid by health care professionals at the scene of an accident or sudden injury. It encourages health care professionals to provide medical care within the scope of their training without fear of being sued for negligence.

References

Davis, B. K. (2002). *Phlebotomy: A Customer Service Approach : a Textbook for Developing Phlebotomy and Customer Service Skills.* Albany: Delmar Thomson Learning Press.

Davis, B. K. (2010). *Phlebotomy: From Student to Professional.* Andover: Cengage Learning Press.

DeLaune, S., & Ladner, P. (2010). *Fundamentals of Nursing.* New York: Cengage Learning.

Ernst, D. J. (2005). *Applied Phlebotomy.* Baltimore: Lippincott Williams & Wilkins Press.

Gibson, J. L., Shah, B. M., & Umberger, R. (2013). *Clinical Medical Assisting: An Introduction to the Fundamentals of Practice.* Burlington: Jones & Bartlett Learning.

Hoeltke, L. B. (2013). *The Complete Textbook of Phlebotomy.* Sidney: Delmar Cengage Learning Press.

Kalanick, K. A. (2004). *Phlebotomy Technician Specialist: A Practical Guide to Phlebotomy.* New York: Delmar/Thomson Learning Press.

Lindh, W., Poole, M., Tamparo, C., & Dahl, B. (2010). *Delmar's Clinical Medical Assisting.* New York : Delmar Cengage Learning Press.

McCall, R. E., & Tankersley, C. M. (2003). *Phlebotomy Exam Review.* Philadelphia: Lippincott Williams & Wilkins Press.

Medtexx Medical Corporation. (2007). *Fundamentals of Phlebotomy .* Retrieved from http://www.depts.ttu.edu/hess/_documents/mccomb/lab_safety/phlebotomy.pdf

National Healthcareer Association Phlebotomy Study guide

Prince, L. G. (2011). *The Art of Phlebotomy.* Bloomington: AuthorHouse Press.

Ridley, J. (2011). *Essentials of Clinical Laboratory Science.* New York : Cengage Learning Press.

Rodak, B. F. (2007). *Hematology: Clinical Principles and Applications.* Philadelphia: Saunders Press.

Strasinger, S. K., & Lorenzo, M. S. (2011). *The Phlebotomy Textbook.* Philadelphia: Davis Co Press.

Turgeon, M. L. (2005). *Clinical Hematology: Theory and Procedures.* Philadelphia: Lippincott Williams & Wilkins Press.

Section One Practice Questions

1. In Urinalysis, what does the MA look for in the urine?
   a. Color
   b. Clarity
   c. Gravity
   d. All of the above

2. Which of the following is used to screen for specific substances?
   a. pH strips
   b. Reagent strips
   c. Drug tests
   d. Melanoma tests

3. Which of the following is also known as the bright-field microscope?
   a. Simple microscope
   b. Spectral microscope
   c. Compound microscope
   d. None of the above

4. The eyepiece is also called:
   a. The ocular
   b. The looking glass
   c. The magnifying glass
   d. The lens

5. Which part of the microscope pivots and allows the lens to rotate?
   a. The base
   b. The nosepiece
   c. The slide
   d. None of the above

6. What is rated by the focal length of the lens?
   a. Objective lens
   b. Spectral lens
   c. Ocular lens
   d. Base lens

7. How is magnification of the low power lens determined?
   a. Focal length of the lens
   b. Multiplying the magnification of the ocular lens by the magnification of the objective lens
   c. Dividing the magnification of the ocular lens by the magnification of the objective lens
   d. None of the above

8. What is the basic unit of length used in lab measurements?
   a. Liter
   b. Meter
   c. Gram
   d. Yard

9. What is the basic unit of weight used in lab measurements?
   a. Liter
   b. Pound
   c. Gram
   d. Yard

10. What is the basic unit of volume used in lab measurements?
    a. Liter
    b. Gram
    c. Ounce
    d. Yard

11. Gram positive bacteria appears:
    a. Deep red
    b. Deep blue
    c. Deep violet
    d. Deep Green

12. Gram negative bacteria appears:
    a. Red
    b. Blue
    c. Violet
    d. Black

13. What is it called when a thin film of specimen is placed into a slide for observation?
    a. A cross section
    b. A sample
    c. A smear
    d. A swab

14. When a thick specimen is received it can be observed by:
    a. Placing it between two slides then pulled apart
    b. Swabbing a sample of it and smearing it onto a slide
    c. Cutting out a cross section and placing it on a slide
    d. Any of the above

15. When should a slide be heat-fixed?
    a. Before the slide is stained
    b. After the slide is stained
    c. During the staining process
    d. None of the above

16. The staining process involves sequential application of:
    a. stain mordant
    b. decolorizer
    c. counterstain
    d. All of the above

17. The gram stain checks for which of the following?
    a. Form

b. Morphology

c. Size

d. All of the above

18. What prevents gram positive bacteria from being affected by alcohol?

a. Peptidoglycan layer and teichoic acids

b. Chloroplasts and granulated reticulum

c. Endothelial endocardiospasms

d. All of the above

19. Gram negative bacteria is affected by alcohol because:

a. Alcohol penetrates the cell wall

b. Alcohol damages the outer membrane

c. Alcohol reacts with the plasma in the membrane

d. Alcohol does not penetrate the cell membrane

20. Which of the following is not a part of the gram stain process?

a. Mordar

b. Decolorizer

c. Counterstain

d. Dye

21. Which of the following is not a good place to take a smear from?

a. Genitalia

b. Open wound

c. Mouth

d. Hair

22. Which of the following statements is false?

a. A smear can be made directly from the swab

b. A smear can be from any body opening

c. A smear can be made from the swab designated for the culture

d. Always wear universal precautions when handling lab samples

23. Which of the following is the proper way to prepare a smear?

a. Rub the swab back and forth several times across the slide

b. Smear or roll the swab across the slide in one direction

c. Roll the slide across the slide both vertically and horizontally

d. Use your finger to spread the specimen across the slide

24. Hematuria is:

a. Excess proteins in the urine

b. Passage of large volumes of urine

c. Absence of urine

d. Presence of blood in urine

25. Anuria is:

a. Excess proteins in the urine

b. Passage of large volumes of urine

c. Absence of urine

d. Presence of blood in urine

26. Polyuria is:
    a. Excess proteins in the urine
    b. Passage of large volumes of urine
    c. Absence of urine
    d. Presence of blood in urine

27. Proteinuria is:
    a. Excess proteins in the urine
    b. Passage of large volumes of urine
    c. Absence of urine
    d. Presence of blood in urine

28. Which of the following should be placed on the label of the urine specimen?
    a. Date and time of collection
    b. Patient's name
    c. Type of specimen
    d. All of the above

29. Which of the following is most commonly used for routine urinalysis?
    a. Sterile sample
    b. First morning sample
    c. Clean catch specimen
    d. Mid-stream specimen

30. Which of the following urinalysis may require catheterization?
    a. Sterile sample
    b. First morning sample
    c. Clean catch specimen
    d. Mid-stream specimen

31. Which specimen is preferred and tends to be the clearest?
    a. Sterile sample
    b. First morning sample
    c. Clean catch specimen
    d. Mid-stream specimen

32. Which specimen is thought to best represent the contents of the bladder?
    a. Sterile sample
    b. First morning sample
    c. Clean catch specimen
    d. Mid-stream specimen

33. Which of the following does urinalysis check?
    a. Specific gravity
    b. Odor
    c. Assessing the volume
    d. All of the above

34. Chemical analysis of urine involves checking for:
    a. pH balance
    b. Urobilinogen
    c. Nitrite
    d. All of the above

35. The microscopic examination for the urine specimen looks at:
    a. Liquid of the urine
    b. Sediment in the urine
    c. Composition of the sample
    d. pH balance

36. Most healthy patients have a urine pH of:
    a. 4.0
    b. 5.0
    c. 6.0
    d. 7.0

37. A normal pH range for fresh urine is:
    a. 2 to 4.0
    b. 3 to 6.5
    c. 4.5 to 8.0
    d. 6.0 to 9.0

38. White blood cells in the urine can be a strong indicator of:
    a. Pregnancy
    b. Urinary tract infection
    c. Glucose
    d. Enzymatic disorder

39. The most common urine test is:
    a. Glucose
    b. Bacterial test
    c. Pregnancy
    d. None of the above

40. Hemoccult Fecal occult blood test tests:
    a. Fecal matter
    b. Blood in the urine
    c. Bacteria in the throat
    d. All of the above

41. A sputum specimen is taken from:
    a. Nostril
    b. Throat
    c. Tear duct
    d. Respiratory tract

42. Which of the following tells the patient about risks, expected outcomes, and alternatives?
    a. Informed consent

b. Consent forms

c. Negligence

d. Admittance paperwork

43. Which of the following is not one of the D's of negligence?
    a. Damage: wrongful activity
    b. Derelict: Breach of duty
    c. Drops: dropping the patient
    d. Duty: Duty of care

44. Which of the following is not an example of tort?
    a. HIPAA
    b. Invasion of privacy
    c. Defamation of character
    d. Battery

45. Which of the following is not required by OSHA in relation to the sharps log?
    a. Type of device used during incident
    b. Color of the sharp container
    c. Department/location of incident
    d. Explanation of the incident

46. Viscera refers to:
    a. Tissues
    b. Organs
    c. Cranial matter
    d. Lungs

47. Systems refer to:
    a. Certain types of tissues
    b. Digestive tract
    c. Collection of cells working together
    d. Group of organs working together

48. Which system effects changes through the pancreas and thyroid?
    a. Immune
    b. Endocrine
    c. Reproductive
    d. Urinary

49. Which system includes ovaries and testes?
    a. Integumentary
    b. Nervous
    c. Reproductive
    d. Endocrine

50. Which system protects the body with skin, hair, and nails?
    a. Integumentary
    b. Immune
    c. Endocrine

d. Cardiovascular

51. Which system involves transporting oxygen throughout the body?
    a. Immune
    b. Nervous
    c. Cardiovascular
    d. Respiratory

52. Which system involves eliminating wastes through the kidneys?
    a. Urology
    b. Reproductive
    c. Nervous
    d. Cardiovascular

53. How many cavities does the body have?
    a. 3
    b. 4
    c. 5
    d. 6

54. The dorsal cavities are located:
    a. In the head
    b. In the back
    c. In the front
    d. In the abdomen

55. The abdominal cavity does not contain:
    a. Spleen
    b. Stomach
    c. Lungs
    d. Intestines

56. The pelvic cavity contains:
    a. Bladder
    b. Stomach
    c. Heart
    d. Esophagus

57. Vertical planes that separate the sides from each other?
    a. Horizontal plane
    b. Frontal plane
    c. Sagittal plane
    d. Transverse plane

58. Which plane divides the body into front and back portions?
    a. Horizontal plane
    b. Frontal plane
    c. Sagittal plane
    d. Transverse plane

59. Which plane divides the body horizontally into an upper and lower part?
    a. Horizontal plane
    b. Frontal plane
    c. Sagittal plane
    d. Transverse plane

60. The back side of the body is:
    a. Superior
    b. Posterior
    c. Anterior
    d. Medial

61. Pertaining to the middle or near the medial plane is referred to as:
    a. Superior
    b. Medial
    c. Dorsal
    d. Inferior

62. An object below another structure is referred to as:
    a. Inferior
    b. Medial
    c. Superior
    d. Dorsal

63. An object above another structure is referred to as:
    a. Inferior
    b. Medial
    c. Superior
    d. Dorsal

64. A person lying on his belly is:
    a. Prone
    b. Supine
    c. Medial
    d. Lateral

65. A person laying on his back is:
    a. Prone
    b. Supine
    c. Medial
    d. Lateral

66. Which of the following are part of the musculoskeletal system?
    a. Ligaments
    b. Bones
    c. Tendons
    d. All of the above

67. Which of the following makes up the axial skeleton?
    a. Skull

b. Ribcage

c. Spine

d. All of the above

68. The bone in the upper portion of the leg is a:

a. Long bone

b. Sesamoid bone

c. Flat bone

d. Short bone

69. The bones in the knuckle joints are:

a. Long bone

b. Sesamoid bone

c. Flat bone

d. Short bone

70. The ribs are:

a. Long bone

b. Sesamoid bone

c. Flat bone

d. Short bone

71. The patella is:

a. Long bone

b. Sesamoid bone

c. Flat bone

d. Short bone

72. A small rounded projection of the bone is a:

a. Tuberosity

b. Tubercle

c. Spine

d. Crest

73. A cavity inside of a bone is:

a. Tubercle

b. Crest

c. Sinus

d. Process

74. The knuckle shaped portion of the bone is:

a. Condyle

b. Sinus

c. Process

d. Spine

75. The projection of the bone is:

a. Condyle

b. Spine

c. Sinus

d. Process

76. A groove in the bone is a:
    a. Sulcus
    b. Sinus
    c. Tuberosity
    d. Crest

77. A rounded orifice in the bone is:
    a. Process
    b. Crest
    c. Foramen
    d. Tuberosity

78. Another name for a projection of the bone is:
    a. Tuberosity
    b. Tubercle
    c. Crest
    d. Foramen

79. An immovable joint is called:
    a. Synarthrosis
    b. Diathrosis
    c. Amphiarthrosis
    d. None of the above

80. A slightly moveable joint is called:
    a. Synarthrosis
    b. Diathrosis
    c. Amphiarthrosis
    d. None of the above

81. A freely moveable joint is called:
    a. Synarthrosis
    b. Diathrosis
    c. Amphiarthrosis
    d. None of the above

82. The upper jawbone is called:
    a. Maxilla
    b. Mandible
    c. Lacrimal bones
    d. Frontal bones

83. The lower jawbone is called:
    a. Maxilla
    b. Parietal bone
    c. Mandible

d. Frontal bone

84. The back of the skull is made up of the:
    a. Frontal bone
    b. Ethmoid bone
    c. Parietal bone
    d. Occipital bone

85. The cheekbone is also known as:
    a. Temporal bones
    b. Zygoma
    c. Maxilla
    d. Vomer

86. The neck bones are also called the:
    a. Thoracic spine
    b. Lumbar spine
    c. Cervical spine
    d. Sacral spine

87. The lower back is part of the:
    a. Thoracic spine
    b. Lumbar spine
    c. Cervical spine
    d. Sacral spine

88. The upper back is part of the:
    a. Thoracic spine
    b. Lumbar spine
    c. Cervical spine
    d. Sacrum

89. Ribs number 1 through 7 attach to the sternum and are also known as:
    a. False ribs
    b. Floating ribs
    c. True ribs
    d. Ribcage

90. The ribs attached to the sternum through cartilage are also called:
    a. False ribs
    b. Floating ribs
    c. True ribs
    d. Ribcage

91. Ribs that do not attach to the sternum at all are also called:
    a. False ribs
    b. Floating ribs
    c. True ribs
    d. Ribcage

92. A bone that is crushed or shattered is:
    a. Colles
    b. Complicated
    c. Comminuted
    d. Greenstick

93. A bone that is driven into the end of another bone is called a:
    a. Hairline fracture
    b. Compression fracture
    c. Pathologic fracture
    d. Impacted fracture

94. A fracture that breaks the bone and pierces an organ is called:
    a. Impacted
    b. Complicated
    c. Compression
    d. Comminuted

95. Increasing the angle of the joint is called:
    a. Extension
    b. Flexion
    c. Adduction
    d. Abduction

96. Movement towards the midline is called:
    a. Extension
    b. Flexion
    c. Adduction
    d. Abduction

97. Movement away from the midline is called:
    a. Extension
    b. Flexion
    c. Adduction
    d. Abduction

98. Decreasing the angle of the joint is called:
    a. Extension
    b. Flexion
    c. Adduction
    d. Abduction

99. A traumatic injury to the soft tissue of the joint is called:
    a. Sprain
    b. Twist
    c. Fracture
    d. Bruise

100.   Which of the following systems cover 22 square feet of the body?
   a. Respiratory
   b. Nervous
   c. Integumentary
   d. Musculoskeletal

101.   What is it called when a bone is completely out of place and the subluxation is partially out of joint?
   a. Twist
   b. Dislocation
   c. Fracture
   d. Dissociation

102.   Which of the following is not a layer of the skin?
   a. Dermis
   b. Epidermis
   c. Subcutaneous
   d. Diaphanous

103.   Hair fibers are made up of:
   a. Peptides
   b. Keratin
   c. Nucleotides
   d. Silk

104.   Which of the following contains sebum and minimizes moisture loss?
   a. Sebaceous glands
   b. Sudderiferous
   c. Lunula
   d. All of the above

105.   The white outer part of the eye is also known as:
   a. Ciliary body
   b. Sclera
   c. Retina
   d. Vitreous humor

106.   The colored part of the eye is:
   a. Iris
   b. Retina
   c. Ciliary body
   d. Sclera

107.   The portion of the eye that deflects light rays as they enter the eye:
   a. Iris
   b. Sclera
   c. Cornea
   d. Retina

108.   The surface of the tympanic membrane is part of the:
   a. External ear
   b. Middle ear
   c. Inner ear
   d. Intercranial aperture

109.   The Eustachian tubes and the opening to the mastoid cavity are part of:
   a. External ear
   b. Middle ear
   c. Inner ear
   d. Intercranial aperture

110.   The part of the ear containing the bony labyrinth, cochlea, and semicircular canals is:
   a. External ear
   b. Middle ear
   c. Inner ear
   d. Intercranial aperture

111.   The external meatus is part of:
   a. Nose
   b. Ear
   c. Eye
   d. Skeleton

112.   The sternocleidomastoid muscle is:
   a. The muscle that separates the abdomen from the thoracic cavity
   b. The muscle that separates the upper and lower portions of the neck
   c. The muscle that separates the right and left ventricles
   d. None of the above

113.   The humerus and the _____ are both part of the shoulder.
   a. Scalpel
   b. Femurus
   c. Scapula
   d. Phalanges

114.   The septum is made up of:
   a. Bones and cartilage
   b. Semicircular canals
   c. Submandibular gland
   d. Sternocleidomastoid

115.   The two kinds of sweat glands are:
   a. Endocrine and apicle
   b. Cutaneous and subcutaneous
   c. Lunar and subdural
   d. Apocrine and Eccrine

116.   The white moonlike portion of the nail bed is:
   a. Lunula

b. Cuticla

c. Solula

d. None of the above

117.   Turning outward is also called:

a. Protraction

b. Rotation

c. Eversion

d. Inversion

118.   Turning inward is also called:

a. Protraction

b. Rotation

c. Eversion

d. Inversion

119.   Which of the following are responsible for movement?

a. Muscles

b. Bones

c. Lungs

d. Organs

120.   Tarsals are considered part of:

a. Appendicular skeleton

b. Axial skeleton

c. Mendibular skeleton

d. None of the above

121.   Upper extremities refer to:

a. Humerus

b. Carpals

c. Radius

d. All of the above

122.   How many pairs of ribs does the human body contain?

a. 8 pair

b. 10 pair

c. 12 pair

d. 14 pair

123.   How many vertebrae does the human body contain?

a. 22

b. 26

c. 28

d. 30

124.   The occipital bone has a large hole at the ventral surface called:

a. Foramen magnum

b. Zygoma

c. Lacrimosa

d. Coccyx

125.　　　A minor fracture that appears as a thin line on the x-ray is called:
a. Impacted fracture
b. Complicated fracture
c. Greenstick fracture
d. Hairline fracture

Answers to section One

1. D
2. B
3. C
4. A
5. B
6. A
7. B
8. B
9. C
10. A
11. C
12. A
13. C
14. A
15. B
16. D
17. D
18. A
19. B
20. A
21. D
22. C
23. B
24. D
25. C
26. A
27. A
28. D
29. B
30. A
31. C
32. D
33. D
34. D
35. B
36. C
37. C
38. B

39. C
40. A
41. D
42. A
43. C
44. A
45. B
46. B
47. D
48. B
49. C
50. A
51. D
52. A
53. C
54. B
55. C
56. A
57. C
58. B
59. D
60. B
61. B
62. A
63. C
64. A
65. B
66. D
67. D
68. A
69. D
70. C
71. B
72. B
73. C
74. A
75. D
76. A
77. C
78. A
79. A
80. C
81. B
82. A
83. C
84. D
85. B
86. C
87. B
88. A

89. C
90. A
91. B
92. C
93. D
94. B
95. A
96. C
97. D
98. B
99. A
100.   C
101.   B
102.   D
103.   B
104.   A
105.   B
106.   A
107.   C
108.   A
109.   B
110.   C
111.   A
112.   B
113.   C
114.   A
115.   D
116.   A
117.   C
118.   D
119.   A
120.   A
121.   D
122.   C
123.   B
124.   A
125.   D

Practice Questions Test One of section 2

1) Phlebotomy is collection of blood for:
   a. Curing disease
   b. Blood count
   c. Laboratory analysis
   d. All of the above

2) Phlebotomists are responsible for:
   a. Collecting blood through capillary puncture
   b. Offering high quality care
   c. Collecting blood through venipuncture
   d. All of the above

3) What recent development has increased the national need for Phlebotomists?
   a. An increase nationwide infectious diseases
   b. Flu season
   c. Recent cases of MRSA
   d. The shortage of Registered Nurses

4) Which of the following is not required of a Phlebotomist?
   a. Collecting blood for analysis
   b. Transporting blood for analysis
   c. Quality control
   d. Analyzing the specimen in the lab

5) Which of the following skills are necessary in order to be a successful Phlebotomist?
   a. Communication skills
   b. Knowledge of infection control procedures
   c. Both A and B
   d. None of the Above

6) Students must achieve how many successful venipunctures for certification?
   a. 15
   b. 25
   c. 30
   d. 10

7) Students must achieve how many successful capillary sticks for certification?
   a. 10
   b. 30
   c. 25
   d. 5

8) Students must achieve what on the National Certification Exam?
   a. 70%
   b. 80%
   c. 90%
   d. None of the Above

9) Which of the following techniques will be used in this course?
   a. Vacuum collection

b. Syringe collection

c. Capillary/skin puncture

d. All of the above

10) Which department would perform a test on formed or cellular elements of the blood?

a. Parasitology

b. Hematology

c. Oncology

d. Nephrology

e. Neuropathy

11) Which department would perform ova and parasite tests on the blood?

a. Parasitology

b. Hematology

c. Oncology

d. Nephrology

e. None of the Above

12) By studying and examining cells, which of the following occurs?

a. Disorders and infections are detected

b. Diagnosis are confirmed

c. Treatment can be instituted and monitored

d. None of the above

e. Both A and C

13) Which of the following is the most common specimen collected for Hematology?

a. Platelets

b. Red blood cells

c. White blood cells

d. Whole blood

e. Plasma

14) Whole blood is usually collected in a tube with:

a. An orange top and LMNO anti-coagulant

b. A blue top

c. A lavender top with EDTA anti-coagulant

d. A green top with sodium citrate

15) Which of the following is not part of the chemistry section of the lab

a. Electrophoresis

b. Globular Reticulation

c. Toxicology

d. Immunochemistry

16) The coagulation section of the laboratory usually analyses what?
    a. Complete profiles
    b. Toxins
    c. Cell regeneration
    d. Hemostasis

17) The blood bank is responsible for all except:
    a. Collection
    b. Storage
    c. Analysis
    d. Preparation for transfusion

18) Which of the following is not a part of the Laboratory?
    a. Blood Bank
    b. Serology
    c. Urinalysis
    d. Microbiology
    e. Oncology

19) Which section would be responsible for growing cultures and checking for microorganisms?
    a. Blood Bank
    b. Microbiology
    c. Urinalysis
    d. Nephrology

20) Which section would check for antibodies in order to search for the presence of microorganisms?
    a. Microbiology
    b. Serology
    c. Oncology
    d. Urinalysis
    e. Blood bank

21) Which of the following organs does not form blood in the body?
    a. Heart
    b. Spleen
    c. Thymus
    d. Lymph Nodes

22) Which of the following organs do form blood in the body?
    a. Liver
    b. Lymph Nodes
    c. Spleen
    d. Both B and C

e.   Both A and C

23) Which of the following is transported by the blood?
   a.   Oxygen
   b.   Calcium
   c.   Water
   d.   Potassium

24) Which of the following excretes toxins from the blood?
   a.   Kidney
   b.   Lungs
   c.   Liver
   d.   Skin
   e.   All of the above

25) Choose the true statement from the following:
   a.   Veins allow blood to flow away from the heart
   b.   Arteries allow blood to flow to the heart
   c.   Capillaries connect veins to arteries
   d.   Arteries connect capillaries to veins
   e.   Veins connect capillaries to arteries

26) Choose the true statement from the following:
   a.   Arteries allow blood to flow away from the heart
   b.   Capillaries are the same thing as venules
   c.   Veins allow blood to flow towards the heart
   d.   Both A and C
   e.   Both A and B

27) Choose the false statement from the following:
   a.   Blood is composed of a liquid part which is plasma
   b.   Arteries are thick walled to enable them to withstand pressure
   c.   Capillaries divide the heart into cavities
   d.   The circulatory system is divided into two parts

28) Blood is circulated through the lungs for enrichment with Oxygen and:
   a.   Enrichment with iron
   b.   Removal of Carbon Dioxide
   c.   Removal of iron
   d.   A fiber scrub

29) The skin is made up of all of the following except:
   a.   Epidermis
   b.   Dydimus

c. Dermis

d. Fatty Tissue

30) The function of the circulatory system is to:

    a. Deliver Oxygen and nutrients

    b. Remove hormones and enzymes

    c. Expel toxins from the body

    d. Protect the body

31) Which of the following is true?

    a. The heart acts as two pumps in series

    b. Pulmonary circulation carries deoxygenated blood from the lungs into the right ventricle

    c. Each side of the heart has one chamber and two valves

    d. The aortic valve is a lunar valve between the right ventricle and the aorta

32) The tricuspid valve is what?

    a. An atrioventricular valve

    b. A semi-lunar valve

    c. A capillary

    d. A ventricle

33) The pulmonic valve is located where?

    a. The left ventricle and the pulmonary artery

    b. The inferior vena cava

    c. The circle of Willis

    d. the right ventricle and the pulmonary artery

    e. None of the above

34) Which of the following is not a layer of the heart?

    a. The Myocardium

    b. The Endocardium

    c. The Triocardium

    d. The Epicardium

35) Which of the following is not a blood vessel?

    a. Vein

    b. Venule

    c. Artery

    d. Arteriole

    e. All of the above are blood vessels

36) Which of the following are composed only of a layer of endothelial cells?

    a. Arteries

b. Capillaries

c. Veins

d. Venules

e. Vena Cava

37) How many liters of blood does the average adult contain?

    a. 1-2

    b. 3-4

    c. 5-6

    d. 7-8

    e. 9-10

38) Plasma does not contain which of the following?

    a. Nucleotides

    b. Proteins

    c. Electrolytes

    d. Hormones

    e. Gases

39) What percent of plasma is made up of water?

    a. 75%

    b. 87%

    c. 92%

    d. None of the above

40) Formed elements makes up what percentage of blood?

    a. 25%

    b. 45%

    c. 65%

    d. 75%

41) Which of the following formed blood cells comprises 99% of formed elements in blood?

    a. Erythrocytes

    b. Thrombocytes

    c. Leukocytes

    d. Hemoglobin

    e. Reticulocytes

42) Which of the following formed cells are also known as white blood cells?

    a. Erythrocytes

    b. Thrombocytes

    c. Leukocytes

    d. Hemoglobin

e. Reticulocytes

43) Which of the following white blood cells engulf and digest bacteria?
   a. Neutrophils
   b. Lymphocytes
   c. Monocytes
   d. Basophils
   e. Eosinophils

44) Which of the following carry histamine?
   a. Neutrophils
   b. Monocytes
   c. Eosinophils
   d. Lymphocytes
   e. Basophils

45) Which of the following are active against parasitic infections?
   a. Lymphocytes
   b. Eosinophils
   c. Basophils
   d. Monocytes
   e. Neutrophils

46) Which of the following are active against viruses?
   a. Eosinophils
   b. Basophils
   c. Monocytes
   d. Lymphocytes
   e. Neutrophils

47) Which white blood cells transform into macrophages when they cross from the blood into tissue?
   a. Eosinophils
   b. Monocytes
   c. Leukocytes
   d. Neutrophils
   e. Basophils

48) Thrombocytes are also known as:
   a. Granules
   b. Basophils
   c. Antibodies
   d. Platelets

49) Thrombocytes are small irregularly shaped packets of what?
   a. Cytoplasm
   b. Hemoglobin
   c. Megakaryocytes
   d. Histamine

50) The process by which blood vessels are repaired after injury is called what?
   a. Hemostasis
   b. Hematocrit
   c. Electrophoresis
   d. Sedimentation

51) Hemostasis begins as:
   a. Clot formation
   b. Vascular contraction
   c. Platelet plug
   d. Coagulation

52) Fibrinolysis is:
   a. A test used to evaluate the extrinsic pathway
   b. The breakdown and removal of the clot
   c. A test to evaluate the intrinsic pathway
   d. Primary hemostasis
   e. Used to monitor Coumadin therapy

53) Which site should be checked first for venipuncture?
   a. Basilic veins
   b. Median veins
   c. Antecubital area
   d. Cephalic veins
   e. Brachial veins

54) Which areas should be avoided for venipuncture?
   a. Arms in casts
   b. Areas of scarring
   c. Arm with intravenous infusions
   d. Edematous arms
   e. All of the above

55) Where should the tourniquet be placed?
   a. 2 to 3 inches beneath the proposed site
   b. Directly on top of the proposed site
   c. 2 inches above the propose site
   d. 3 to 4 inches beneath the proposed site

  e. 3 to 4 inches above the proposed site

56) Which fingers could you check the site with?
  a. Thumb or Middle finger
  b. Pinky or Index finger
  c. Middle Finger or Ring finger
  d. Index finger or Middle finger

57) Which of the following is true about veins?
  a. They all run left to right on the arm
  b. Not all veins go up and down on the arm
  c. All veins go up and down on the arm
  d. All above statements are false

58) What should you not puncture?
  a. A vein that travels horizontally across the arm
  b. A vein that travels vertically across the arm
  c. A vein that pulsates
  d. A vein that is round
  e. None of the Above

59) Which vein is considered the vein of choice?
  a. The Cephalic vein
  b. The Median Cubital vein
  c. The Antecubital Fossa
  d. The Basilic vein
  e. The Tortuous vein

60) Which vein is often the only vein that can be palpated in an obese patient?
  a. The Cephalic vein
  b. The Median Cubital vein
  c. The Antecubital Fossa
  d. The Basilic vein
  e. The Sclerosed vein

61) Which vein is located near the Brachial artery?
  a. The Cephalic vein
  b. The Median Cubital vein
  c. The Antecubital Fossa
  d. The Basilic vein
  e. The Thrombotic vein

62) Which veins are susceptible to infection and may produce erroneous tests?
  a. The Cephalic vein

b. The Antecubital Fossa

c. Thrombotic veins

d. Sclerosed veins

e. Tortuous veins

63) Hard or cordlike veins are called:

a. Sclerosed veins

b. Thrombotic veins

c. Sclerosed veins

d. Tortuous veins

64) Which of the following is true?

a. If it is possible you should always draw blood from an arm with a running IV

b. If it is possible you should always draw blood from Tortuous veins

c. If it is possible you should always draw blood from the Antecubital Fossa

d. If it is possible you should always draw blood from the Brachial artery

e. If it is possible you should always draw blood from an A-V fistula sight

65) Which of the following is not a method of venipuncture?

a. The vacuum method

b. The butterfly method

c. The IV method

d. The syringe method

e. All of the above are proper methods

66) Which method transfers blood to a vacuum tube?

a. The vacuum method

b. The butterfly method

c. The syringe method

d. All of the above

67) Which of the following should you have before you perform the venipuncture?

a. Laboratory requisition slip

b. Nurse's approval

c. Betadine

d. Morphine

68) Which of the following is not a kind of antiseptic?

a. Povidone-iodine

b. Chlorhexidine gluconate

c. Dihydrogen monoxide

d. Alcohol

69) Which gauge is the smallest needle in diameter?

a. 18 gauge

b. 23 gauge

c. 16 gauge

d. 20 gauge

70) Which gauge is the smallest used for drawing blood?

    a. 16 gauge

    b. 23 gauge

    c. 20 gauge

    d. 18 gauge

71) A winged infusion set might be used in which of the following scenarios?

    a. A normal patient with veins that can be palpated

    b. An obese patient with veins that can be palpated

    c. A pediatric or elderly patient

    d. All of the above would require a winged infusion set

    e. None of the above would use a winged infusion set

72) Which of the following can be used to prevent a venous outflow of blood?

    a. A latex strip

    b. A blood pressure cuff

    c. Tourniquet with Velcro

    d. All of the above

73) Which of the following supplies would you need for obtaining a specimen?

    a. Gloves

    b. Vacutainer tubes

    c. A mask

    d. Both A and C

    e. Both A and B

74) If blood cannot be obtained what options are acceptable?

    a. Probe the vein

    b. Attempt a second venipuncture

    c. Ask the doctor to do it for you

    d. Attempt as many punctures as is needed to get the job done

75) Which of the following is the most common complication of phlebotomy procedure?

    a. Hematoma

    b. Hemoconcentration

    c. Fainting

    d. Phlebitis

    e. Septicemia

76) Which of the following is inflammation of the vein with formation of a clot?
   a. Petechiae
   b. Thrombus
   c. Hematoma
   d. Thrombophlebitis
   e. Trauma

77) Which of the following is inflammation of the vein as a result of repeated venipuncture on that vein?
   a. Hemoconcentration
   b. Septicemia
   c. Fainting
   d. Petechiae
   e. Phlebitis

78) Which of the following is a result of leaving the tourniquet on too long increasing the proportion of formed elements to plasma?
   a. Thrombus
   b. Fainting
   c. Hemoconcentration
   d. Petechiae
   e. None of the above

79) Which of the following are tiny red spots from rupturing capillaries?
   a. Petechiae
   b. Hemoconcentration
   c. Thrombophlebitis
   d. Thrombus
   e. All of the above

80) Which of the following could potentially alter test results?
   a. Collecting blood from an arm with a running IV in it
   b. Collecting blood from edematous tissue
   c. Faulty technique
   d. Extended tourniquet time
   e. All of the above

81) When does quality control begin?
   a. Before collection
   b. During collection
   c. After collection
   d. In the lab

82) Which of the following may alter test results before collection?
   a. Faulty technique

b. Rimming clots

c. Inadequate fast

d. Failure to invert tubes

83) Which of the following may alter test results after collection?
   a. Under filling tubes
   b. Medication interference
   c. Faulty techniques
   d. Improper use of serum separator

84) Which of the following may alter test results during collection?
   a. Patient posture
   b. Failure to invert tubes
   c. Processing delays
   d. Poor coordination with other treatments

85) What piece of equipment has a small opening at one end that connects to the needle, and a wide opening at the other end for the collection tube?
   a. Winged infusion sets
   b. Vacutainer needles
   c. Needle adaptors
   d. Tourniquets

86) When recapping a needle:
   a. Hold the cap in one hand and the needle with the other hand
   b. Never recap without a safety device
   c. Hold the cap with your teeth and the needle with your hand
   d. Only cap a needle that is small

87) Which antiseptic is most commonly used?
   a. Iodine pad
   b. 40% Isopropyl alcohol pad
   c. 70% Isopropyl alcohol pad
   d. None of the above

88) The antecubital area is:
   a. The area on the back of the hand
   b. The area behind the knee
   c. The forearm
   d. The bend of the upper arm

89) Which phase of coagulation creates a stable fibrin clot?
   a. Fibrinolysis phase
   b. Coagulation phase

    c. Platelet phase

    d. Vascular phase

90) Which of the following is the upper chamber of the heart?

    a. Atrium

    b. Ventricle

    c. Valve

    d. Myocardium

91) Which organs receive cellular waste from the blood for excretion?

    a. Liver and Gallbladder

    b. Kidneys and Gallbladder

    c. Lungs and Liver

    d. Lungs and Intestines

    e. All of the above

92) What is responsible for the formation of blood cells?

    a. The Liver

    b. Bone Marrow

    c. The Heart

    d. The Lungs

93) Which layer of muscle is the contractile element of the heart?

    a. Myocardium

    b. Epicardium

    c. Endocardium

    d. All of the above

94) The capillaries are composed of:

    a. Myocardium

    b. Epithelial cells

    c. Endocardium

    d. Squamous cells

    e. Epicardium

95) Which of the following is responsible for forming blood clots?

    a. Red blood cells

    b. White blood cells

    c. Hemoglobin

    d. Platelets

96) Which of the following can be caused by introducing a pathogenic organism during venipuncture?

    a. Phlebitis

    b. Thrombus

c. Petechiae

d. Septicemia

97) Which of the following will not alter test results?

a. Patient misidentification

b. Failure to wear gloves

c. Improper use of serum

d. Processing delays

98) Syncopy is another name for:

a. Hematoma

b. Thrombocytosis

c. Edema

d. Fasting

e. Fainting

99) Which of the following is an avoidable injury caused by probing?

a. Hematoma

b. Phlebitis

c. Thrombophlebitis

d. Trauma

100)   Which of the following should a phlebotomist ask before attempting venipuncture?

a. Whether the patient requires medication

b. Whether the patient has been fasting

c. Whether the patient is dehydrated

d. Whether the patient needs a band-aid

Answers to Test One of section 2

1) C

2) B

3) D

4) D

5) C

6) B

7) A

8) A

9) D

10) B

11) A

12) E

13) D

14) C

15) B

16) D

17) C

18) E

19) B

20) B

21) A

22) D

23) A

24) E

25) C

26) D

27) C

28) B

29) B

30) A

31) A

32) A

33) D

34) C

35) E

36) B

37) C

38) A

39) C

40) B

41) A

42) C

43) A

44) E

45) B

46) D

47) B

48) D

49) A

50) A

51) B

52) B

53) C
54) E
55) E
56) D
57) B
58) C
59) B
60) A
61) D
62) E
63) A
64) C
65) C
66) D
67) A
68) C
69) B
70) B
71) C
72) D
73) D
74) B
75) A
76) D
77) E
78) C
79) A
80) E
81) A
82) C
83) D
84) B
85) C
86) B
87) C
88) D
89) B
90) A
91) D
92) B
93) A
94) B
95) D
96) D

97) B
98) E
99) D
100) B

Multiple Choice questions Test Two of section 2

1) Outpatients should sit for _____ to ensure recovery from venipuncture?
   a. 10 minutes
   b. 15 minutes
   c. 20 minutes
   d. 25 minutes
   e. 30 minutes

2) When should you release the tourniquet and immediately remove the needle?
   a. If the vein rolls upon attempted venipuncture
   b. If a hematoma begins to develop
   c. If the venipuncture begins to swell during the process
   d. None of the above

3) The first step of the venipuncture process is to:
   a. Verify the requisition for the tests
   b. Palpate the antecubital fossa
   c. Explain the procedure to the patient
   d. Identify the patient

4) While checking the patient's ID you must check the ID number and:
   a. Have him/her to state his/her name
   b. Have him/her extend the arm for the venipuncture
   c. Palpate the vein for venipuncture
   d. None of the above

5) Which of the following will aide in engorging the vein?
   a. Having the patient raise his/her hand over the head
   b. Moving the patient into a reclining position
   c. Having the patient make a fist
   d. Tightening the tourniquet
   e. All of the above

6) The tourniquet should be applied where?
   a. 2-3 inches below the puncture site
   b. 3-4 inches below the puncture site
   c. 2-3 inches above the puncture site
   d. 3-4 inches above the puncture site
   e. None of the above

7) When should the tourniquet be applied?
   a. Before initially palpating the vein
   b. Before gathering the necessary equipment
   c. Before identifying the patient
   d. Before checking the requisition orders
   e. Before palpating the vein while looking for the straightest point

8) When should you assemble the needle holder
   a. While palpating the vein
   b. While tying the tourniquet
   c. While the antiseptic is drying
   d. While the patient is making a fist
   e. Any of the above

9) How should you anchor the vein?
   a. By tying the tourniquet and slightly pulling back the skin
   b. By placing your thumb below the antecubital area and slightly pulling back the skin
   c. By doing a second venipuncture and anchoring the vein to the muscle below
   d. Any of the above

10) Which direction should the bevel face?
   a. Up
   b. Down
   c. Away from the patient's body
   d. Towards the patient's body

11) What angle should the needle enter the puncture site?
   a. 5-10 degrees
   b. 10-25 degrees
   c. 15-30 degrees
   d. 20-40 degrees

12) Once blood begins to flow:
   a. Remove the needle
   b. Palpate the vein
   c. Release the tourniquet

    d. Put on gloves

13) When filling the tubes:
    a. Follow order of the draw
    b. Ask patient to verbally state name and birthday
    c. Have the patient make a fist
    d. Palpate the vein

14) What should be placed over venipuncture site before removing the needle?
    a. A glove
    b. Alcohol prep pad
    c. Nothing
    d. Gauze

15) In order to stop the bleeding:
    a. Have patient bend his/her arm
    b. Apply pressure with your fingers
    c. Have patient stand up
    d. Tighten the tourniquet

16) Which of the following must be written on the collected specimen?
    a. Patient ID number
    b. Date and time
    c. Your initials
    d. All of the above

17) When should you call for help?
    a. If the bleeding does not stop after two minutes
    b. If the bleeding does not stop after three minutes
    c. If the bleeding does not stop after 5 minutes
    d. If the bleeding does not stop after 8 minutes

18) When should the specimen be labeled?
    a. Before entering the room
    b. After collection
    c. Before putting on gloves
    d. After exiting the room

19) What should be done with the used sharps?
    a. They should be left for the nurse to clean up
    b. They should be placed in the biohazards sharps container
    c. They should be placed in the biohazards transport bag
    d. They should be used on the next patient

20) What is done after the bleeding stops?
    a. Gauze is placed over the venipuncture site
    b. Sharps are discarded
    c. Adhesive bandage is applied over a gauze square
    d. Tourniquet is released

21) When you fail obtain blood after a puncture what should you do first?
    a. Remove the needle and try again
    b. Rotate the needle by a half turn
    c. Use a different needle
    d. None of the above

22) When a phlebotomist fails to obtain blood, he/she may need to do all except:
    a. Move the needle back a little
    b. Rotate the needle by a half turn
    c. Probe with the needle
    d. Push the needle in a little further

23) Which of the following may be a reason that blood is not obtained?
    a. Insufficient vacuum in the tube
    b. Bevel of the needle resting against the vein wall
    c. Tube slipping out of the holder
    d. All of the above

24) Which of the follow could be a reason that a tube might have insufficient vaccum?
    a. It is a non-vacuum tube
    b. It has a very fine crack
    c. It has a defect
    d. Both A and B
    e. Both B and C

25) You are tending to a patient and suspect that the patient has a collapsed vein. Which of the following should you do?
    a. Choose another vein and use a butterfly or a syringe
    b. Reposition the needle and use the same vacuum tube
    c. Probe the site and try again
    d. Any of the above

26) When there is an order for a fasting test, who should verify with the patient that he/she has fasted?
    a. The nurse
    b. The doctor
    c. The phlebotomist
    d. The lab tech

27) Which of the following would a timed test be used for?
   a. Determining blood levels of medication
   b. To evaluate frequent low blood sugar
   c. To check for microorganisms
   d. To evaluate diabetes mellitus

28) A two hour postprandial test would be used for:
   a. Determining blood levels of medication
   b. To test glucose tolerance
   c. To evaluate diabetes mellitus
   d. To monitor changes in the patient's condition
   e. All of the above

29) The PKU test would be used for:
   a. Checking for microorganisms
   b. To detect Phenylketonuria
   c. To evaluate diabetes mellitus
   d. To evaluate low blood sugar

30) Who would be most likely to receive a PKU test?
   a. A cancer patient
   b. An infant
   c. An obese patient
   d. A middle aged man
   e. A flu patient

31) Cold Agglutinins are formed in response to which illness?
   a. Influenza
   b. Acute RSV
   c. Myocardial Infarction
   d. Atypical Pneumonia
   e. All of the above

32) Which of the following is not true about testing for Cold Agglutinins?
   a. The antibodies formed may attach to red blood cells at temps below body temp
   b. The specimen must be kept warm until the serum is separated
   c. Blood is collected in red topped tubes pre-warmed in incubators
   d. Tubes are pre-warmed at 37 degrees Celsius for approx. 30 minutes
   e. All above statements are true

33) Which of the following test requires a chilled sample?
   a. Parathyroid hormone
   b. Arterial blood gases
   c. PKU

d. A and B

e. A and C

34) What should be done in order to keep a blood sample chilled?

    a. Place in a dry cooler

    b. Place on dry ice

    c. Place on crushed ice

    d. Keep at room temperature

35) Which of the following is not a light sensitive test?

    a. Bilirubin

    b. Arterial blood gas

    c. Porphyrins

    d. Beta Carotene

36) In order to protect a sample from light, what should you do?

    a. Wrap sample in aluminum foil

    b. Place sample in pocket

    c. Place sample in dry cooler

    d. Get it to the lab as soon as possible

    e. All of the above are acceptable

37) Dermal puncture collects blood from:

    a. Arteries

    b. Arterioles

    c. Capillaries

    d. Veins

    e. Venules

38) Which of the following is used to perform a dermal puncture?

    a. Scalpel

    b. hypodermic needle

    c. Butterfly set

    d. Lancet

39) When should a dermal puncture be performed?

    a. When there is a need for a large amount of serum

    b. When there is a lack of hypodermic needles

    c. When venipuncture is inadvisable

    d. When the patient is a child

40) Which statement is false?

    a. A lancet has a predetermined depth of puncture

    b. Heel punctures for infants should not exceed 2.0 mm

c. Dermal punctures can be done on infants and adults

d. It is acceptable to use an adult lancet on a pediatric patient

41) Where should a heel puncture be performed?

    a. On a previous puncture site

    b. On the back of the heel

    c. On the arch of the foot

    d. On the heel of the hand

    e. On the plantar surface of the heel

42) Where should a dermal puncture be performed on adults and non-infants?

    a. On the heel slightly to the side of the lines of the footprint

    b. On the distal segment of the third or fourth finger

    c. On the pinky finger in the center of the fingerprint lines

    d. On the medial segment of the third or fourth finger

43) After identifying the patient and assembling the equipment you should:

    a. Use a lancet to puncture the site

    b. Check requisition orders

    c. Clean site with 70% isopropyl alcohol

    d. Prepare puncture device

    e. Warm the site

44) Which of the following is essential for collecting specimens for PH or blood gases with dermal puncture?

    a. Keeping the specimen in the dark

    b. Placing the specimen on ice

    c. Keeping the specimen warm

    d. Warming the puncture site

    e. All of the above are essential

45) Which of the following would be a good candidate for dermal puncture?

    a. A person with fragile veins

    b. An infant

    c. A person with inaccessible veins

    d. A person who is obese

    e. All of the above

46) Which of the following is an example of additive carryover?

    a. Medications in the blood affecting the lab results

    b. Iodine or Alcohol from the skin contaminating the results

    c. Coagulant from one tube getting into another specimen tube

    d. All of the above are examples

47) Which of the following statements is false?
   a. The tops of the collection tubes are not sterile
   b. Medication that a patient has taken may interact with additives
   c. Wrong order of draw may lead to cross-contamination
   d. Blood cultures should be collected before other tubes are filled

48) Which of the following tubes should be filled first?
   a. Tubes for blood cultures
   b. Tubes containing EDTA
   c. Tubes containing sodium citrate
   d. Serum tubes

49) Which of the following tubes should be filled last?
   a. Tubes for blood cultures
   b. Tubes containing EDTA
   c. Tubes containing sodium fluoride
   d. Tubes with clot activators
   e. Any of the above

50) Which of the following would be the correct order for filling tubes?
   a. Blood cultures, sodium citrate, heparin, EDTA
   b. Heparin, sodium citrate, EDTA, blood cultures
   c. EDTA, sodium citrate, blood cultures, heparin
   d. sodium citrate, blood cultures, EDTA, heparin
   e. All of the above are acceptable

51) Which of the following would be the correct order for filling tubes?
   a. Blood cultures, serum tubes, sodium fluoride, sodium citrate
   b. Serum tubes, sodium fluoride, sodium citrate, blood cultures
   c. Sodium fluoride, serum, blood cultures, sodium citrate
   d. Blood cultures, sodium citrate, serum, sodium fluoride
   e. None of the above

52) Which of the following could render the tube of specimen useless?
   a. Cracks in the tubes
   b. Expired tubes
   c. Microclots
   d. Defects in the tube
   e. All of the above

53) When you are in doubt you should:
   a. Ask the nurse
   b. Choose a different tube
   c. Read the label

d. Perform the test anyway

54) Which of the following is a way that a phlebotomist may contract an infection?
    a. Inhalation
    b. Needle sticks
    c. Direct contact
    d. All of the above

55) Which of the following is not a way to prevent infection spread?
    a. Wearing gloves
    b. Proper hand washing
    c. Isolating infected body substances
    d. All of the above

56) Which of the following is true about medical asepsis?
    a. It eliminates risk of infection spread
    b. It aims at destroying pathologic organisms
    c. It is necessary to use on all patients
    d. All of the above

57) Chain of infection is defined as:
    a. Links, each of which is necessary for disease to spread
    b. The method of which an infectious agent leaves its reservoir
    c. Infectious microorganisms that can be classified into groups
    d. None of the above

58) Which of the following is not an agent of infection?
    a. Virus
    b. Fungi
    c. Host
    d. Parasite
    e. bacteria

59) Which of the following is not part of the chain of infection?
    a. Portal of exit
    b. Agents
    c. Parasites
    d. Mode of transmission

60) Which of the following must be interrupted in order to break the chain of infection?
    a. Portal of exit
    b. Agents
    c. Mode of transmission

d. Any of the above

61) Which of the following is an example of droplet transmission?
    a. Contracting an illness when a co-worker sneezes
    b. Contracting an illness from contact with blood
    c. Contracting an illness by touching a surface
    d. Contracting an illness from a mosquito bite

62) Which of the following is an example of contact transmission?
    a. Contracting an illness when a co-worker sneezes
    b. Contracting an illness from contact with blood
    c. Contracting an illness from drinking parasitic water
    d. Contracting an illness from a mosquito bite

63) Which of the following on a human body could be a portal of exit?
    a. The liver
    b. The spleen
    c. The mouth
    d. The stomach

64) Which of the following on the human body could be a portal of entry?
    a. Smooth, unbroken skin
    b. Veins
    c. Arterioles
    d. Mucous membranes

65) Which of the following allows the infectious agent into a susceptible host?
    a. Portal of entry
    b. Portal of exit
    c. Agents
    d. Mode of transmission

66) Which of the following patients best represents a susceptible host?
    a. A teenager coming in for a sports physical
    b. A child coming in for a school physical
    c. An baby coming in for a well child checkup
    d. A premature infant

67) Which of the following is an example of medical asepsis?
    a. Hand washing
    b. Disinfecting a room
    c. Using Iodine on a proposed venipuncture site
    d. All of the above

68) Which of the following is an example of barrier protection?
   a. Hand washing
   b. Disinfecting a room
   c. Wearing gloves
   d. All of the above

69) Which of the following is an example of barrier protection?
   a. Goggles
   b. Face shields
   c. Gloves
   d. All of the above

70) Which of the following is meant to prevent direct contact with blood and body fluids?
   a. Transmission-based precautions
   b. Standard precautions
   c. Barrier precautions
   d. Basic precautions
   e. None of the above

71) Which of the following is not a standard precaution?
   a. Wearing gloves
   b. Recapping a sharp
   c. Wearing a mask
   d. All are standard precautions
   e. None are standard precautions

72) Which patient would you use transmission-based precautions for?
   a. A patient coming in for a physical
   b. A patient with heart problems
   c. A patient with tuberculosis
   d. A patient with a broken arm
   e. All of the above

73) Which of the following are types of transmission-based precautions?
   a. Contact precautions
   b. Airborne precautions
   c. Droplet precautions
   d. All of the above

74) Which of the following would prevent microorganisms from being dispersed widely by air currents?
   a. Contact precautions
   b. Airborne precautions
   c. Droplet precautions
   d. All of the above

e. B and C only

75) Which of the following would prevent contamination from large particle droplets?
   a. Contact precautions
   b. Airborne precautions
   c. Droplet precautions
   d. All of the above
   e. B and C only

76) Which of the following would prevent contamination from physical transfer?
   a. Contact precautions
   b. Airborne precautions
   c. Droplet precautions
   d. All of the above
   e. B and C only

77) Which department is responsible for identifying and minimizing workplace hazards?
   a. OSHA
   b. NSA
   c. ASHO
   d. NASA
   e. Security

78) What types hazards are identified workplace hazards?
   a. Biologic
   b. Sharps
   c. Chemical
   d. Electrical
   e. All of the above

79) Which of the following is an example of a physical workplace hazard?
   a. Bunsen burners
   b. Cleaning agents
   c. Wet floors
   d. Lancets
   e. Fungi

80) Which of the following is an example of a biological workplace hazard?
   a. Glass on the floor
   b. Exposed electrical wires
   c. Heavy lifting
   d. Wet floors
   e. Mold on the walls

81) A coworker has slipped on the floor and broken an arm. You should:
   a. Apply pressure
   b. Elevate the arm
   c. Set the arm
   d. Get help

82) Which of the following is not a symptom of shock?
   a. Rapid, weak pulse
   b. Deep breathing
   c. Expressionless, staring eyes
   d. Pale, clammy skin

83) When a person is in shock you should not do which of the following?
   a. Call for assistance
   b. Keep the victim warm
   c. Have the patient stand up
   d. Maintain an open airway
   e. All of the above are good remedies for shock

84) Which of the following is essential for maintaining good legal practices?
   a. Practicing confidentiality
   b. Giving information to all family members
   c. Doing whatever it takes to get the blood drawn
   d. All of the above are good legal practices

85) When a patient refuses a blood draw a phlebotomist should:
   a. Attempt to draw blood using restraints
   b. Ask the nurse for help holding down the patient
   c. Explain why the test is important
   d. All of the above
   e. None of the above

86) When a patient refuses a blood draw after an explanation, a phlebotomist should:
   a. Attempt to draw blood using restraints
   b. Notify the appropriate people and document the refusal
   c. Explain a second or third time why the test is important
   d. All of the above are acceptable

87) Which of the following is not an element of negligence?
   a. Duty of care
   b. Derelict of duty
   c. Direct cause of injury
   d. Damage

e. Draining of assets

88) Which of the following protects people rendering aid at the scene of an accident or injury?
   a. Healthcare provider protection act
   b. First responder laws
   c. Good Samaritan laws
   d. None of the above

89) Which of the following is not a common cause for tort in the healthcare field?
   a. Invasion of privacy
   b. Rendering aid
   c. Battery
   d. Defamation of character

90) What must you have before releasing patient information to a third party?
   a. A requisition order
   b. A doctor's order in the chart
   c. Written consent from the third party
   d. Verbal consent from the patient
   e. Written consent from the patient

91) Which of the following should not be used to cleanse and prepare an area for venipuncture?
   a. 1:10 bleach solution
   b. Iodine
   c. Isopropyl alcohol
   d. All of the above are good cleansing choices

92) In order to avoid lawsuits:
   a. Never perform a procedure against the patient's wishes
   b. Never release information to a third party without written consent
   c. Never perform a procedure that you are not certified for
   d. Never do any of the above

93) Who is most at risk for exposure to blood and body fluids?
   a. Healthcare workers
   b. Patients
   c. Family of patients
   d. Family of healthcare workers

94) What are the reasons that you should wear gloves?
   a. To minimize risk of transferring microorganisms from patient to patient
   b. To provide a protective barrier
   c. To reduce the likelihood of infecting the patient with a microorganism

d. All of the above

95) Which of the following is an example of portal of entry?
    a. Liver
    b. Patella
    c. Mucous membranes
    d. Ventricles

96) Why should dermal puncture be used on infants?
    a. Because infants cry
    b. Because infants squirm
    c. Because infants' veins are small and difficult to locate
    d. Because infant heels are most convenient

97) Dermal puncture is not suitable for which of the following tests?
    a. Blood cultures
    b. PKU tests
    c. Bilirubin tests
    d. All are suitable for venipuncture

98) When using a blood pressure cuff:
    a. Inflate the cuff all the way
    b. Use a tourniquet in tandem with the cuff
    c. Perform only a dermal puncture
    d. Inflate to between the patient's systolic and diastolic pressure

99) Before performing a venipuncture you should always:
    a. Release the tourniquet
    b. Fill the tubes in order of the draw
    c. Place gauze on the venipuncture site
    d. Introduce yourself

100)   Which of the following is not a vein that you should draw blood from?
    a. The antecubital
    b. The jugular
    c. The cubital
    d. The medial
    e. Any of the above are suitable for venipuncture

Answers to Test Two

1) B
2) C
3) A
4) A
5) C
6) D
7) E
8) C
9) B
10) A
11) C
12) C
13) A
14) D
15) B
16) D
17) D
18) B
19) B
20) C
21) B
22) C
23) D
24) E
25) A
26) C
27) A
28) C
29) B
30) B
31) D
32) E
33) D
34) C
35) B
36) A
37) C
38) D
39) C
40) D
41) E
42) B
43) E
44) D

45) E
46) C
47) B
48) A
49) C
50) A
51) D
52) E
53) C
54) D
55) D
56) B
57) A
58) C
59) C
60) D
61) A
62) B
63) C
64) D
65) A
66) D
67) D
68) C
69) D
70) B
71) B
72) C
73) D
74) B
75) C
76) A
77) A
78) E
79) C
80) E
81) D
82) B
83) C
84) A
85) C
86) B
87) E
88) C

89) B
90) E
91) A
92) D
93) A
94) D
95) C
96) C
97) A
98) D
99) D
100)   B

OTHER TITLES FROM THE SAME AUTHOR:

1. Phlebotomy Test Prep Vol 1, 2 & 3

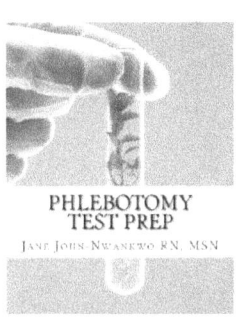 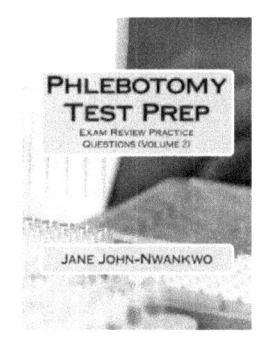 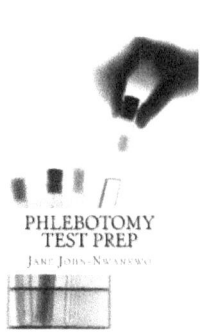 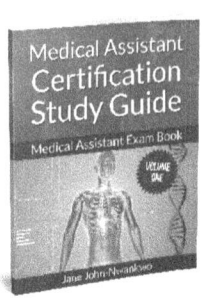

2. Work At Home Jobs For Nurses & Other Healthcare Professionals

3. CNA Exam Prep: Nurse Assistant Practice Test Questions. Vol. One and Two

4. Patient Care Technician Exam Review Questions: PCT Test Prep

5. Medical Assistant Certification Study Guide Volume 1

6. Medical Assistant Test Preparation

7. EKG Test Prep

8. Nurses' Romance Series

9. The Home Health Aide Textbook

10. Medical Administrative Assistant Exam Prep

And Many More Books You Would Like!

Visit www.healthcarepracticetest.com NOW!

OTHER TITLES FROM THE SAME AUTHOR:

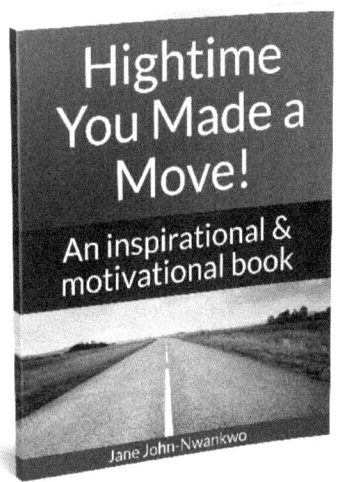

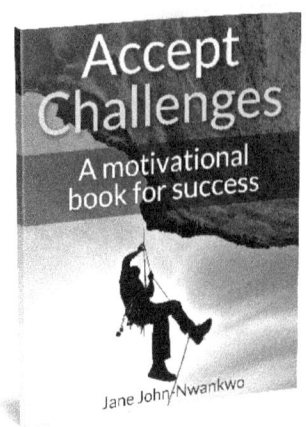

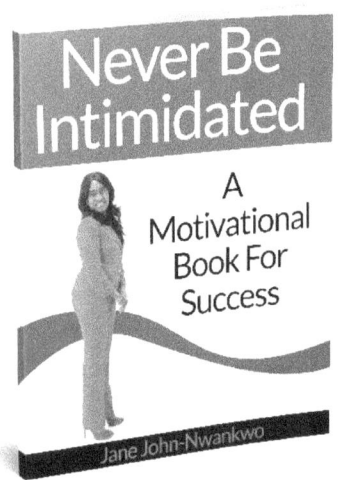

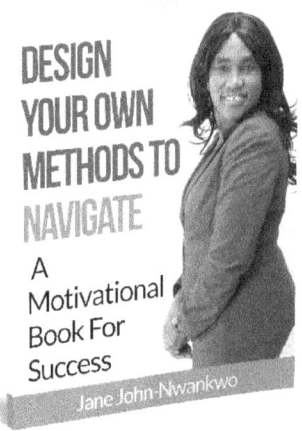

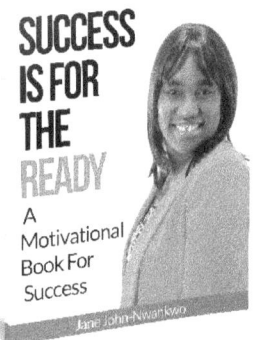

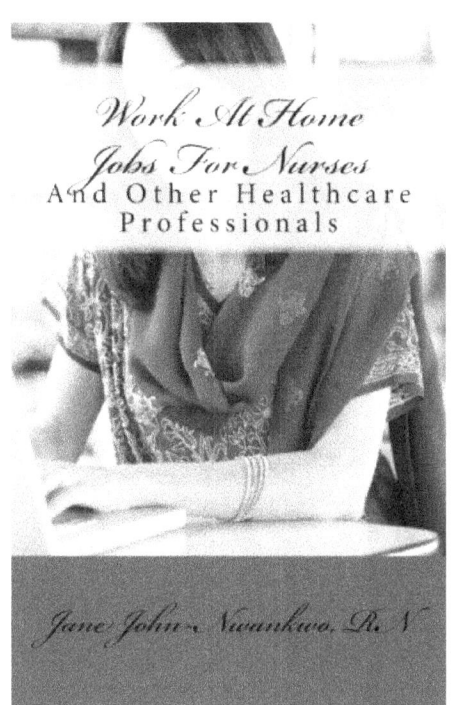

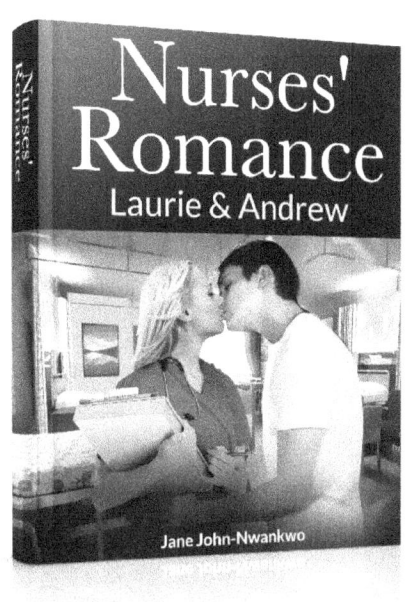

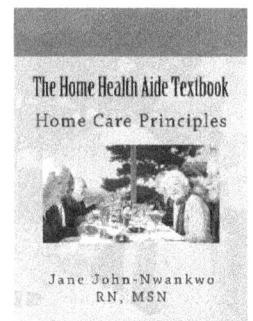

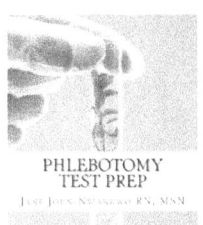

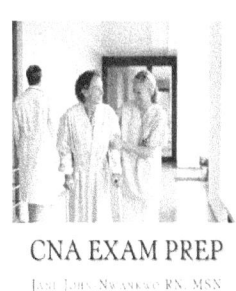

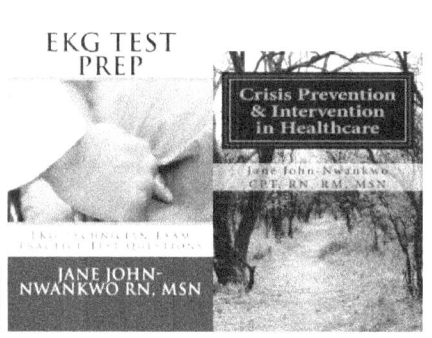

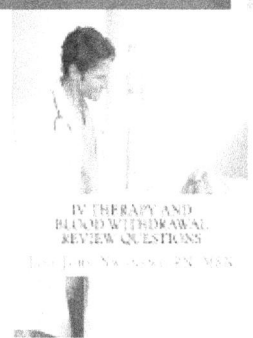

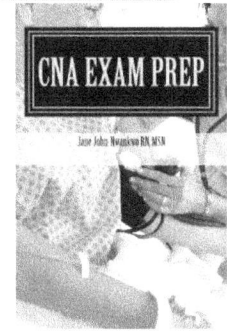

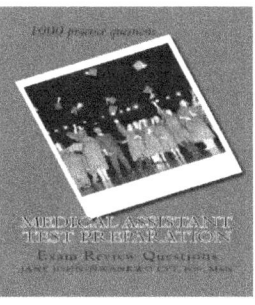

www.ingramcontent.com/pod-product-compliance
Lightning Source LLC
Chambersburg PA
CBHW080259180526
45167CB00006B/2587